Understanding Sickle Cell Disease

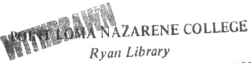

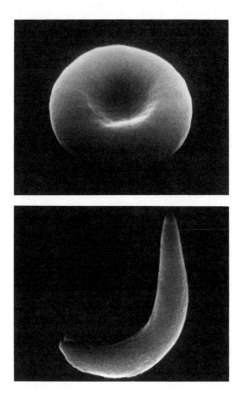

Photomicrographs of red blood cells from a sickle cell patient. When surrounded by a high oxygen concentration, red blood cells look normal (top). When oxygen is depleted, the cells assume a distorted, or "sickle," shape (bottom). Photomicrographs courtesy of Dr. James White (University of Minnesota School of Medicine).

Understanding Sickle Cell Disease

Miriam Bloom, Ph.D.

Understanding Health and Sickness Series
University Press of Mississippi
Jackson

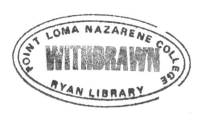

Copyright © 1995 by the University Press of Mississippi
All rights reserved
Manufactured in the United States of America
98 97 96 95   4 3 2 1
The paper in this book meets the guidelines for permanence and dura-
bility of the Committee on Production Guidelines for Book Longevity
of the Council on Library Resources.

Illustrations by Regan Causey

Library of Congress Cataloging-in-Publication Data
Bloom, Miriam.
    Understanding sickle cell disease / Miriam Bloom.
        p.   cm. — (Understanding health and sickness series)
    Includes bibliographical references and index.
    ISBN 0-87805-744-7. — ISBN 0-87805-745-5 (pbk.)
    1. Sickle cell anemia—Popular works. I. Title.
    II. Series.
RC641.7.S5B56   1995
616.1'527—dc20   94-44275
                                CIP

British Library Cataloging-in-Publication data available

Contents

Acknowledgments

I am indebted to Dr. Martin Steinberg (University of Mississippi School of Medicine and Jackson Veterans Affairs Medical Center) for critically reviewing this entire manuscript and for sharing a great deal of information. Dr. J. Clinton Smith (University of Mississippi School of Medicine) critically reviewed Chapters 1 through 4 of my first draft and offered valuable suggestions. Gail Chadwick (Jackson State University) and Dr. Helen Barnes (University of Mississippi School of Medicine) critically reviewed the section on family planning (Chapter 6). Dr. Stephanie Bloom (University of California College of Medicine, San Francisco) gave me a private mini-course in sickle cell disease and followed it up (as always) with thoughtful suggestions.

Introduction

Our understanding of sickle cell disease and our management of sickle cell patients have improved enormously in the past two decades. Modern medical care is permitting people with the disease to live longer, more comfortable, and more productive lives. Genetic counseling and advanced family-planning techniques offer couples at risk of having sickle cell children a choice in the matter, and laboratory scientists are moving closer to a cure.

About 1 out of 375 Americans of African descent is born with sickle cell disease, as is a smaller fraction of Americans descending from families from the Mediterranean area, the Middle East, and India. In addition, about 8 percent of black Americans who do not suffer from the disease itself carry a gene for it that can be transmitted to their children. Some of these individuals know that they carry the gene; others do not.

This book was written for all people interested in sickle cell disease—for those who have the disease, for their families, for carriers of the sickle cell gene, for teachers, and for those who want to update and round out their information. Sickle cell disease bears enormous biological, social, and historic importance, and it has captured the interest of physicians and scientists since sickle cells were first described in medical literature almost a century ago.

We begin this book with a brief overview of sickle cell disease and then lead you through the way the sickle cell gene is inherited. The inheritance patterns of the disease are diagrammed so that you can determine a couple's chance of having sickle cell children. Next comes an explanation of why the sickle cell gene is so common in certain groups of people, but so rare in others. We discuss the relationship between the sickle cell gene and its geographic origins and how the gene was spread throughout history, including the modern slave-trading era.

Next, we take a closer look at the red blood cell and pinpoint the molecule that causes the trouble—*hemoglobin S*. We relate important discoveries about hemoglobin S and the effect this abnormal hemoglobin has on the cells that carry it. Following this discussion, we present a medical overview of sickle cell disease in both children and adults. We tell about the variety of symptoms individuals may suffer and why, and we discuss the problems of pregnancy. In addition, we talk about the emotional aspects of the disease, which play an important role in family and school settings. The discussion of the nature of sickle cell disease is followed by a chapter on the care of people who have it, emphasizing the home situation. We distinguish between the symptoms that can be handled at home and those that say, "Head for the hospital." Pain and drugs are dealt with. Next, we tell how it is possible in the United States today for couples carrying sickle cell genes to raise families that are free of sickle cell disease. More is known about sickle cell disease than about any other inherited disease, yet no cure exists. There is little doubt, however, that one will ultimately be devised. In the final chapter, we survey current research efforts and the promise they hold.

Many sources were consulted during the writing of this book. Two publications regularly drawn from were *Sickle Cell Disease* by Graham Serjeant (second edition, Oxford University Press, 1992) and *Sickle Cell Disease: Basic Principles and Clinical Practice,* edited by Stephen Embury, Robert Hebbel, Narla Mohandas, and Martin Steinberg (Raven Press, 1994). Much of the information for Chapter 5 (How to Care for People with Sickle Cell Disease) came from *A Parent's Handbook for Sickle Cell Disease,* edited by Shellye Lessing and Elliott Vichinsky (State of California Department of Health Services, Genetic Disease Branch, 1991).

Understanding Sickle Cell Disease

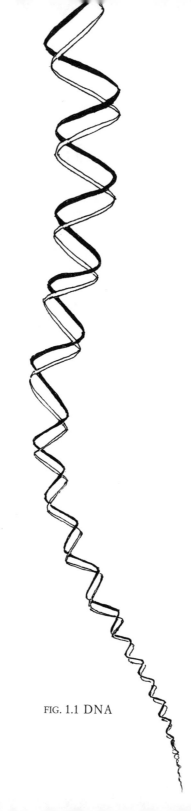

FIG. 1.1 DNA

1. Sickle Cell Disease and How It Is Inherited

There are many different causes of human disease. These include malnutrition, infection, radiation, physical injury, and mistakes in body chemistry. Sickle cell disease, an inherited disease, is caused by a mistake in body chemistry. Sickle cell disease is the result of abnormal *hemoglobin*, the oxygen-carrying molecule of the red blood cell. The disease affects all parts of the body, but it does not affect everyone in the same way. Sickle cell disease differs widely from one individual to another. It differs in both the extent of its complications and its severity. Proper medical care coupled with a good home-support system can alleviate symptoms, prolong life, and help sickle cell people to be active and productive.

People born with sickle cell disease cannot outgrow it. People who are not born with sickle cell disease can never get it. It is not contagious, and it is not caused by anything we do or anything we come in contact with. *Sickle cell trait* runs in the same families as sickle cell disease, but people with sickle cell trait do not have sickle cell disease, and they never will. In some instances, however, they can have children who do. People with sickle cell disease have inherited two damaged *genes* (units of heredity), one from each parent. The parents inherited the damaged genes from their parents, who inherited them from their parents, and so on, going back hundreds of generations. Genes are like blueprints. They carry information, not on blue paper, but in long chemical strands called DNA that twist around each other to form a *double helix* (fig. 1.1). When these chemicals are damaged, the information they carry is changed, and it remains changed forever. In sickle cell disease, it is the genes for hemoglobin that are damaged, and that is why the hemoglobin is abnormal.

Hemoglobin's job is to pick up oxygen in the lungs and release it to other parts of the body. The problem with sickle cell hemoglobin is that often it cannot get to other parts of the body. The way hemoglobin gets around the body is by being carried inside red blood cells. The blood, pumped by the heart, travels through the circulatory system. Blood leaving the heart is carried in arteries. Blood returning to the heart is carried in veins. Connecting the arteries and veins is a series of smaller, branching vessels that are often narrower than the red blood cell itself. The red blood cell, therefore, must squeeze through these tiny vessels.

Red blood cells from normal individuals have no problem squeezing through the tiny vessels. Inside these red cells, the hemoglobin is dissolved in a watery solution. It remains dissolved under all conditions—whether there is lots of oxygen around or only a little, for example. Thus, the normal red blood cell is always soft and flexible enough to squeeze through vessels narrower than itself. Inside the red blood cell of a person with sickle cell disease, however, the hemoglobin stays dissolved under some conditions, but under others, it comes out of solution. Instead of remaining liquid, it forms crystals that twist the red cell out of shape. When this happens, the red cell is no longer soft and flexible and it cannot squeeze through small vessels. In addition, the hemoglobin crystals damage the red cell membrane. These things—the crystallized hemoglobin and the damaged red blood cell membrane—have the following consequences:

1. Since the red blood cells cannot squeeze through small blood vessels, the vessels become clogged and blood flow backs up. Oxygen does not get delivered to the organs that need it.

2. When an organ has its oxygen supply cut off, it is damaged and it produces pain. The damage can be serious and the pain can be severe.

3. When red blood cells are damaged, the body destroys

them. So many red cells are damaged and destroyed in people with sickle cell disease that they suffer from chronic anemia.

4. People with sickle cell disease are not robust. They are in danger of getting infections, they are frequently incapacitated, they do not grow and develop as well as their peers, and they are not likely to live as long.

Although sickle cell disease is found in several groups of people, it is most prevalent among people of African ancestry. Over 50,000 black Americans suffer from sickle cell disease, which makes it a major public health concern in the United States.

How Sickle Cell Disease Is Inherited

Sickle cell disease runs in families. It is transmitted from one generation to the next in classic, well-understood, patterns. Once it is known whether a couple carries genes for sickle cell disease, the likelihood of their children being born with it can be predicted. People who do not know whether they carry sickle cell genes can call their local health department, their regional network for genetics services, or their state genetic services coordinator (see Appendix) and ask where they can be tested.

In sickle cell disease, normal hemoglobin, *hemoglobin A* (*Hb A*), is replaced by sickle cell hemoglobin, *hemoglobin S* (*Hb S*). Other blood conditions leading to different types of sickle cell disease are sometimes inherited together with Hb S. These include *hemoglobin C* (*Hb C*) and *beta thalassemia*. Hb C is another abnormal hemoglobin. It is found primarily among people from West Africa. In beta thalassemia, the amount, rather than the kind of hemoglobin, is abnormal. It is found primarily among people from around the Mediterranean Sea. That, in fact, is how the disease got its name—*thalassa* is the Greek word for sea. People who have one Hb S gene and one Hb A gene have sickle cell trait. They do not have sickle cell disease, and their lives are generally normal (see Chapter 4). To understand sickle cell disease inheritance, it is necessary to understand the laws of chance. In fact, all inheritance follows the laws of chance. When a child is conceived, be it a son or a daughter (and the smart money there goes on fifty-fifty odds), each parent makes an equal contribution to the child's genetic makeup. That is, one half of each parent's genes becomes one half of the child's genes. Which half is transmitted to the child, however, rests entirely with chance.

Genes are chemicals that carry information. One unit of information is carried by each gene. The information includes instructions for making all of the body's proteins. Some of these proteins serve as the building materials of the body, others serve as *enzymes*, the molecules that make things happen in living systems. By telling cells which proteins to make, genes determine the stuff we are made of, how our bodies grow and develop, and ultimately, all we can become.

Genes come in pairs and are borne on paired *chromosomes*,[1] which are located in their own compartment of the cell, the *nucleus*. Each member of a gene pair is called an *allele*. All the cells that carry genes, except the *gametes* (egg cells and sperm cells), carry one set of maternal genes and one set of paternal genes. Every physical characteristic—from the shape of our ears to the way our gut digests food—is influenced by at least one such allelic pair. When gametes are formed from parental cells, every gene pair separates, and one of the alleles (the maternal or the paternal, depending on the luck of the draw) goes into each gamete. Thus, each gamete gets a completely different set of genes, all decided by chance. The egg cell receives a complete unpaired set of genes and the sperm cell receives a complete unpaired set of genes. At conception (the union of an egg and a sperm) (fig. 1.2), genes again become paired. This process has two important results:

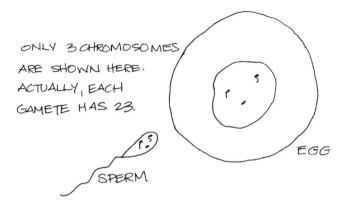

FIG. 1.2 At conception, egg and sperm cells each contribute an equal number of chromosomes.

1) One half of the child's genes will come from the father (via the sperm), and one half will come from the mother (via the egg). This is true even when the child resembles one parent more than it resembles the other.

2) Each parent will contribute half of his or her own genes to the child. There is no telling, however, what mix of genes (which genes from the parent's mother and which from the parent's father) will be in that half.

At conception, the male normally releases about 150 million sperm cells (on that basis alone, any one of us could have been 150 million others of us). Each sperm cell, therefore, has about a 1-to-150-million chance of being the one that fertilizes an egg. If there is an egg. The odds of there being a receptive egg varies each day of the menstrual cycle for fertile women, from very low to very high.

Since the human *genome* (complete set of chromosomal genes) contains perhaps 100,000 genes, and each is paired, the chance of ending up with one specific set of genes is similar to the chance of ending up with one specific sequence of heads and tails when you flip 100,000 coins. Thus, the genome we inherit from our fathers is like the result of 100,000 fifty-fifty chance events, and the genome we inherit from our mothers is like the result of another 100,000 fifty-fifty chance events. In actuality, however, genes are not inherited all that independently. Because genes sit on chromosomes, they are very often inherited together with other genes on the same chromosome. Nevertheless, this is a good way to picture the inheritance of any one gene. The chance of inheriting any particular gene, including the Hb S gene, is fifty-fifty, which is identical to the chance of getting heads (or tails) in a coin flip.

The female coin flips. Heads, the egg gets the mother's allele for type A blood; tails, the egg gets her allele for type B blood (assuming the mother has these genes in the first place). Heads, the egg gets her allele for Hb S; tails, the egg gets her allele for Hb A. Heads, heads, heads, the mother transmits musical, near-sighted, and short-height genes. Tails, tails, tails, she transmits tone-deaf, eagle-eye, basketball-player genes. The father flips, too, and at conception, his genes influencing blood type, hemoglobin, musical ability, eyesight, height, and everything else meet up with the mother's genes, and all the child's potential characteristics are determined at that instant.

A big difference exists between some of the examples of inherited traits listed above and the others. Blood types are absolute; they are determined by genes alone and cannot be changed by the way we live our lives. The genes for musical and athletic ability, on the other hand, only confer potentials; to fulfill them, the corresponding skills must be developed by hard work. Without the inherited potential, however, no amount of hard work will turn someone into a concert violinist or a basketball champion. Eyesight and height are also inherited as potentials; their expression, like the expression of musical and athletic ability, is influenced by how our bodies are nourished, cared for, and used. A boy may be born with the ability to become a great opera star, but if he becomes a smoker, he may never even get into a church choir. Nothing at all, however, short of genetic manipulation (Chapter 7), can influence inherited blood and hemoglobin types. What they are is what they will always be.

Although each parent makes an equal contribution to the child's heredity, not all genes have an equal effect. Some genes are *dominant*. That is, they mask the presence of other, *recessive*, genes. For certain traits, such as A and B blood types, each parental gene is equally influential (*codominant*). If an infant receives a type A gene from its mother and a type B gene from its father (or vice versa), its blood type will be AB. But other genes do not express themselves this way. For example, people who inherit genes for blue eyes from one parent and genes for brown eyes from the other parent do not have blue-brown eyes, nor do they have one blue eye and one brown eye.[2] They usually have two brown eyes. This is because the brown-eye genes cause so much pigment to be made that you cannot even tell that the blue-eye genes (which do not know how to make brown eye pigment) are there. Thus, brown-eye genes are dominant over blue-eye genes. Blue eyes may be the result of a *mutation* (an altered gene). It may be that blue eyes appear blue because the genes that tell the eye how to make brown pigment are defective.

If blue eyes result from a mutation, it is a harmless one. Many mutations, however, are not harmless. More than 2,000 human diseases, including sickle cell disease, are known to be caused by mutations in single genes. Another 2,000 are suspected to be. Sickle cell disease occurs when both copies of a single gene—a hemoglobin gene—are altered. Instead of providing the blueprint for Hb A, either they both provide the blueprint for Hb S, or one provides the blueprint for Hb S and the other provides the blueprint for some other hemoglobin abnormality, such as Hb C or beta thalassemia.

As was mentioned above, when one hemoglobin gene carries the sickle cell mutation and the other hemoglobin gene is normal, people have sickle cell trait. With sickle cell trait, the genes can be viewed as either codominant or recessive, depending on whether we are looking at the hemoglobin or at the disease. If we are looking at the hemoglobin, we see both Hb S and Hb A, so the genes are codominant because their effects are equally apparent. If we are looking at the disease, however, we see someone who appears perfectly healthy, so the sickle cell gene is recessive because it does not cause disease. This is like brown-eye genes masking blue-eye genes; enough Hb A is produced to mask the Hb S, so people with sickle cell trait enjoy normal health.

Now let's try some predictions. We will look at matings between couples with Hb S genes and Hb A genes and see what kind of children they will have. The term "normal" is used in the following exercise to mean that both of the hemoglobin genes are Hb A genes. Here are all the possible kinds of matings:

1. Both parents have sickle cell disease.
2. One parent has sickle cell disease and the other has sickle cell trait.
3. One parent has sickle cell disease and the other is normal.
4. Both parents have sickle cell trait.
5. One parent has sickle cell trait and the other is normal.
6. Both parents are normal.

The diagrams below should help with the analysis of these matings. The top row shows the two possible hemoglobin genes the gametes—eggs or sperm—from one parent can transmit, and the left column shows the two possible hemoglobin genes the gametes—sperm or eggs—of the other parent can transmit, all with equal probability. The boxes at the intersection of the two gamete types show which hemoglobin genes the child from that conception will have. Remember that these genes are sex-neutral; they exert the same effect no matter which parent transmits them.

	CASE 1	
	S	S
S	SS	SS
S	SS	SS

Both parents have sickle cell disease. Since sickle cell disease is recessive, both parents must have two copies of the Hb S gene (or else they would not have the disease). So no matter which gametes combine to form the child, the results will be the same— every child of this mating will receive one Hb S gene from its mother and one Hb S gene from its father. All children born to this couple will have sickle cell disease.

	CASE 2	
	S	S
A	AS	AS
S	SS	SS

One parent has sickle cell disease and the other has the trait. The parent with sickle cell disease has Hb S genes only. Therefore, all of its gametes will have a Hb S gene. The other parent, however, has one Hb S gene and one Hb A gene. The odds of that parent transmitting either gene are equal, or fifty-fifty. For this couple, therefore, two types of conception are equally probable—one between two gametes carrying Hb S genes, and one between a gamete carrying a Hb S gene and a gamete carrying a Hb A gene. All children born to this couple will display either sickle cell disease or sickle cell trait, with the odds being fifty-fifty for each.

	CASE 3	
	S	S
A	AS	AS
A	AS	AS

One parent has sickle cell disease and the other is normal. All the gametes of the sickle cell parent will carry a Hb S gene, and all the gametes of the normal parent will carry a Hb A gene, so all children will inherit one normal and one sickle cell gene. All children born to this couple will have sickle cell trait.

CASE 4	A	S
A	AA	AS
S	SA	SS

Both parents have sickle cell trait. Both parents have an equal chance of transmitting either gene. Half of the time one parent will transmit a Hb S gene, and this will have an equal chance of combining with another Hb S gene from the other parent or with a Hb A gene from the other parent. The other half of the time the first parent will transmit a Hb A gene, and this, too, will have an equal chance of combining with a Hb S gene from the other parent or a Hb A gene from the other parent. Adding these up, we see that 25 percent of these chance events will lead to the union of a Hb S gene with another Hb S gene, 50 percent will lead to the union of a Hb S gene with a Hb A gene, and 25 percent will lead to the union of a Hb A gene with another Hb A gene. Children born to this couple will have a 25 percent chance of having sickle cell disease, a 50 percent chance of carrying sickle cell trait, and a 25 percent chance of being normal.

CASE 5	A	S
A	AA	AS
A	AA	AS

One parent has sickle cell trait and the other is normal. Half of the gametes of the parent with sickle cell trait will carry the Hb S gene, and half will carry the Hb A gene. Since all the gametes of the other, normal, parent will carry a Hb A gene, half of the conceptions will result in a union of a Hb S gene with a Hb A gene, and half will result in a union of two Hb A genes. All the children of this couple will either display sickle cell trait or be normal; the chances are fifty-fifty for each.

CASE 6

	A	A
A	AA	AA
A	AA	AA

Both parents are normal. Neither parent has a sickle cell gene to transmit. All children of this couple will be normal. This will be the case even if the preceding generation (parents of the parents) carried sickle cell genes.

It is important to understand that the probability of having a child with sickle cell disease is the same at every conception. If the probability of conceiving a child with sickle cell disease is 50 percent, it does not mean that 50 percent of the children will have the disease, although that is the most likely outcome. Nor does it mean that the second child will be normal if the first was born with the disease, or vice versa. A 50 percent probability means that every child conceived has a 50 percent likelihood of being born with the disease.

What Is a Gene?

The knowledge we have today on what genes are and how they work is profound, dazzling, and powerful. But genetics did not even exist as a science until 1865 (the year slavery was abolished in the United States), when Gregor Mendel, an Austrian monk with a scientific turn of mind, published his studies on inheritance in the edible pea. It was Mendel who discovered genes. He discovered also that they exist in pairs, that one of each pair is randomly transmitted by each parent to its offspring, that genes are not changed by being inherited, and that their effect is the same whether the male or the female parent transmits them. This pattern of inheritance, which is the pattern of inheritance for sickle cell disease, is called *Mendelian inheritance.* Genes carry the blueprints for our bodies (and for the bodies of all other living things) in a special code. Genes are made of *deoxyribonucleic acid*, or DNA. DNA, a chemical that you can mush around in a test tube, determines the structure (and therefore the function) of living things by encoding the proteins that the living things are made of. And since genes are inherited, they must also know how to duplicate themselves. How DNA duplicates itself and encodes information, and how proteins are made from the code, have been revealed in a series of stunning research achievements. One of the most important of these was the discovery of the structure of DNA, which was accomplished at Cambridge University by James Watson and Francis Crick in 1953. This discovery launched the modern era of molecular biology, and, therefore, our understanding of sickle cell disease.

Genes, then, have two vital roles: They duplicate themselves for transmission from one generation to the next, and, by directing the manufacture of the body's proteins, they determine how living things are made and how they function.

Proteins, the stuff we are made of, are large molecules made up of *amino acid* chains. Twenty amino acids are used by living systems, and, as humans, we must obtain all twenty from food. We eat animal or vegetable proteins, digest them down to their individual amino acids, and then rebuild these amino acids into the chains that make up our own proteins. The know-how for converting the amino acids we eat into the flesh and enzymes of our own bodies resides in our DNA.

DNA is a linear molecule of variable length that usually exists in a double-stranded state. The two strands form a spiral ladder—that double helix we mentioned before. The sides of the ladder are made of repeating sugar-phosphate units. The rungs of the ladder consist of paired *nucleotide bases* (fig. 1.3). There are four nucleotide bases—*adenine* (A), *thymine* (T), *guanine* (G), and *cytosine* (C). A, T, G, and C are letters of the genetic alphabet. Three letters together form a genetic word. Genetic sentences are constructed from these three-letter

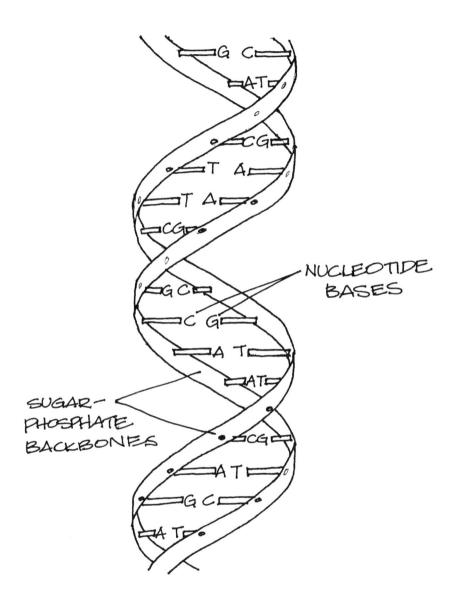

NUCLEOTIDE
BASES

SUGAR-
PHOSPHATE
BACKBONES

FIG. 1.3 The structure of DNA

words (all made up of various sequences of A, T, G, and C). These sentences tell our cells, starting with a fertilized egg, how to make and run our bodies. This, then, is the language of life.

Four letters taken three at a time ("triplets") can form 64 different words. (Try it.) The 64 words formed by the genetic alphabet determine the twenty amino acids we eat, plus three punctuation marks ("End the protein here" signals). Subtracting the 3 punctuation marks from the original 64 words leaves 61 words. Since there are 61 possible words but only 20 amino acids for them to represent, it follows that at least some amino acids are represented by more than one word. The language of life has synonyms.

Which amino acid or punctuation mark corresponds to which three-letter word is called the *genetic code*. In a series of ingenious experiments conducted in the early 1960s, Marshall Nirenberg at the National Institutes of Health and his collaborators cracked the genetic code. They used extracts of bacteria (*Escherichia coli*) to make proteins in laboratory dishes. They tested strands of all 64 nucleotide base triplets (which they made themselves), one at a time, to see what amino acid the *E. coli* extract would make in response. Figure 1.4 shows what the code looks like. Later experiments revealed that bacteria and humans and just about all other living things use the same genetic code, making it a universal language, and the oldest language on earth.

Genes, then, are made up of DNA strands. These are long strings of nucleotide bases (A, T, G, and C) attached to a spiral backbone and arranged in specific sequences. Proteins are made up of amino acid chains. The specific sequence of the amino acids in protein chains is determined by the specific sequence of the nucleotide bases in DNA. All living things, be they peas, bacteria, or humans, are unique collections of specific, genetically determined proteins.

Hemoglobin (which contains a total of 574 amino acids) is

SECOND LETTER

FIRST LETTER	U	C	A	G	THIRD LETTER
U	UUU, UUC PHE UUA, UUG LEU	UCU, UCC, UCA, UCG SER	UAU, UAC TYR UAA, UAG STOP	UGU, UGC CYS UGA STOP UGG TRP	U C A G
C	CUU, CUC, CUA, CUG LEU	CCU, CCC, CCA, CCG PRO	CAU, CAC HIS CAA, CAG GLN	CGU, CGC, CGA, CGG ARG	U C A G
A	AUU, AUC, AUA ILE AUG MET	ACU, ACC, ACA, ACG THR	AAU, AAC ASN AAA, AAG LYS	AGU, AGC SER AGA, AGG ARG	U C A G
G	GUU, GUC, GUA, GUG VAL	GCU, GCC, GCA, GCG ALA	GAU, GAC ASP GAA, GAG GLU	GGU, GGC, GGA, GGG GLY	U C A G

ABBREVIATIONS FOR AMINO ACIDS

GLY	GLYCINE
ALA	ALANINE
VAL	VALINE
LEU	LEUCINE
ILE	ISOLEUCINE
SER	SERINE
THR	THREONINE
ASP	ASPARTIC ACID
GLU	GLUTAMIC ACID
LYS	LYSINE

ARG	ARGININE
ASN	ASPARAGINE
GLN	GLUTAMINE
CYS	CYSTEINE
MET	METHIONINE
PHE	PHENYLALANINE
TYR	TYROSINE
TRP	TRYPTOPHAN
HIS	HISTIDINE
PRO	PROLINE

FIG. 1.4 The genetic code

an important and readily available protein molecule and has been the subject of extensive research. In 1940, Irving Sherman, a young medical student at Johns Hopkins University, published his observation that when light was passed through the red blood cells of sickle cell patients, the sickled cells transmitted the light differently than the nonsickled cells. Dr. William Castle, the Harvard professor of medicine who had figured out how pernicious anemia develops, understood the implications of Sherman's observation; it suggested a special orientation of molecules inside the cells. In a chance conversation during a train ride, Castle mentioned Sherman's observation to Linus Pauling,[3] the distinguished chemist at the California Institute of Technology who had worked extensively with hemoglobin. Pauling, assuming that hemoglobin was at the heart of the sickling matter, followed up that chance conversation with experiments that compared hemoglobin samples from normal people, people with sickle cell trait, and people with sickle cell disease. By subjecting the hemoglobin samples to *electrophoresis*, a technique that separates proteins on the basis of their electric charge, Pauling found that he had two different hemoglobins in his samples. Normal individuals had one type, sickle cell disease patients had another, and individuals with sickle cell trait had both types. Pauling concluded, "This investigation reveals, therefore, a clear case of a change produced in a protein molecule by an allelic change in a single gene...."[4] This was the first demonstration of a change in protein structure showing Mendelian inheritance. It is of historic interest that this important discovery came from a study of sickle cell hemoglobin.

But what was this change? What was the abnormality in sickle cell hemoglobin? In 1956, in the same laboratory at Cambridge where Watson and Crick had worked out the structure of DNA, Vernon Ingram set out to answer that question. He used an enzyme to break Hb S and Hb A into smaller pieces, which he then compared by electrophoresis. The two hemoglobins were identical in all but one of those pieces. When he studied that piece further, Ingram discovered that Hb S differed from Hb A in a single amino acid: *valine* was substituted for *glutamic acid* in one position. Here, pinpointed at last, was the thing that made sickle cell hemoglobin different from normal hemoglobin. How this one tiny change causes the symptoms of sickle cell disease is discussed in Chapter 3.

The Genetic Injury in Sickle Cell Disease

In the light of modern molecular genetics, it is possible to figure out the mutation that brought about the change from glutamic acid to valine in the hemoglobin molecule. Locating the genetic code for these two amino acids in figure 1.4, we can compare the two triplets that code for glutamic acid with the four that code for valine:

Genetic Codes

Glutamic Acid	Valine
GAA	GTT
GAG	GTC
	GTA
	GTG

Going through each code reveals the following. In position 1, the two triplets for glutamic acid and the four triplets for valine all have a G, so it is evident that there was no mutation here in going from the code for glutamic acid to the code for valine. In position 2, all glutamic acid codes have an A and all valine codes have a T, so an A-to-T mutation must have occurred in position 2. When we look at position 3, we see that either GAA or GAG could have been the original glutamic acid triplet, because, in either case, only one mutation, a change from A to T in position 2, would have caused a change from a glutamic acid code to a valine code. Thus, the event converting normal adult hemoglobin to sickle cell hemoglobin was most likely a change of A to T in position 2 of either GAA or GAG in a Hb A gene. (Actually, it was a GAG that changed to GTG.) We will see in Chapter 2 that, in human history, this event happened more than once.

As it turns out, more than one gene serves as a blueprint for hemoglobin. Hemoglobin molecules consist of four subunits—two of each of two different protein chains. These are designated the *alpha* and *beta chains*. Since one gene can code for only one protein, two different genes are needed to code for the two different kinds of hemoglobin subunits. The chain responsible for sickle cell hemoglobin is the beta chain. Whereas the sixth amino acid in the beta chain of Hb A is glutamic acid, the sixth amino acid of the beta chain of Hb S is valine. (In Hb C, a mutation in the same place causes the substitution of lysine for glutamic acid as the sixth amino acid. Using figure 1.4, you can determine the mutation that changed Hb A to Hb C.) The beta chain of Hb A is 146 amino acids in length. Therefore, the tiniest of changes—the alteration of just one of the three bases that code for the sixth amino acid of a 146-amino acid sequence—is responsible for sickle cell disease.

Thus, the inheritance of sickle cell disease follows from the two essential features of genes—their ability to encode information and their ability to make copies of themselves. Genes must make copies of themselves or else organisms could not reproduce. Reproduction is characteristic of life, but so is imperfection (as you may have noticed). Genes sometimes make mistakes when they duplicate themselves, and then the information they carry into the next generation is changed. Usually this is lethal. Sometimes, however, the mutation is neutral or even advantageous. In such cases, the new gene becomes part of the population, and it, too, reproduces with fidelity, following the same laws of heredity as its parent, the nonmutant gene. That is how sickle cell disease began. What chance events originally caused the hemoglobin genes to mutate is not known, but we will see in the next chapter why they persisted.

2. Who Has Sickle Cell Disease and Why?

The largest proportion of sickle cell disease cases occurs among blacks, both in Africa and in countries with a slave-trading history. In the United States there is some regional variability. There is a lower frequency of cases in the North than in the South, where isolated pockets of considerably higher frequency have been reported. According to 1993 estimates, over 50,000 African Americans have sickle cell disease, while about one in twelve carries the sickle cell gene.

Whites, too, carry the sickle cell gene, although many people do not realize it, and even a blue-eyed, blonde-haired person can have sickle cell disease. Sickle cell disease occurs among whites from the Middle East, India, and the Mediterranean. The gene is common, for example, among Israeli Arabs, Saudis, Turks, Greeks, Sicilians, and Cypriots. The case that led to the important discovery by Dr. William Castle in 1938 that sickling slows down blood flow (which, in turn, causes more sickling; see Chapter 3) involved a white woman from Cleveland, Ohio, whose family was Italian.

In the United States, most cases of sickle cell disease occur among African Americans, and the earliest published reports of the disease here all involved black patients. Although the Hb S gene is most common in Africa, sickle cell disease went unreported in African medical literature until the 1870s. This may be because the symptoms of the disease were similar to the symptoms of other tropical diseases and because blood was not usually examined. Also, children born with sickle cell disease usually died in infancy, so physicians may not have seen many of them as patients. The tribal populations were all too familiar with sickle cell disease, however, and they created their own

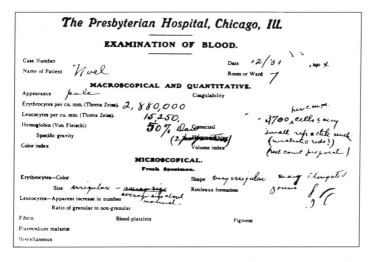

FIG. 2.1 This 1904 report on Walter Clement Noel's blood was written by Dr. Ernest Irons, who was the first physician to describe sickle cells. Note the sketches of the cells in the lower right corner.

names for it. The tribal names all carry repeating syllables (to symbolize repeating painful episodes?): *ahututuo* (Twi tribe), *chwecheechwe* (Ga tribe), *nuidudui* (Ewe tribe), and *nwiiwii* (Fante tribe). In some African tribes, as many as 40 percent of the people carry the sickle cell gene.

In the United States in 1846, a paper titled "Case of Absence of the Spleen" was probably the first to describe sickle cell disease.[5] It discussed the condition in a runaway slave who had been tried and executed for murdering another runaway slave. A physician autopsied the body one hour after the hanging (the court ordered the body to be "delivered to any surgeon who would demand it") and noted the unusual body build of "the unfortunate murderer," the symptoms he had suffered during his lifetime, and "the strange phenomenon of a man having lived without a spleen." Although the slave's condition was typical of sickle cell disease (Chapter 4), the doctor had no way of knowing it because, in his world, sickle cell disease had not yet been discovered.

The first formal report of sickle cell disease—one that included a description of sickle cells—came out of Chicago about a half-century later.[6] In 1910, Dr. James Herrick reported "peculiar elongated and sickle shaped" red blood cells in "an intelligent negro of 20." These sickled cells were discovered by a hospital intern, Dr. Ernest Irons, who examined the patient's blood and sketched the strange cells in his examination write-up (fig. 2.1). In 1922, after three more cases were reported, the disease was named "sickle cell anemia."

The story of that first sickle cell patient's short life has recently been told. He was Walter Clement Noel,[7] the product of a marriage between two wealthy land-owning families in Grenada, West Indies. He came to Chicago in 1904 to study dentistry in one of the best schools in the country, and he was likely to have been the only black student there. (His concerned mother wrote a note to the dean, "I will be very glad if you would take an interest in him, and see that he does his work, especially as he is a stranger.") Despite repeated hospitalizations for his illness, Noel completed his training along with his classmates three years later. He then returned to Grenada and practiced dentistry until he died, at the age of thirty-two, of pneumonia. Dr. Noel is buried in Grenada overlooking the Caribbean in the Catholic Cemetery of Sauters. A stone still marks his grave (fig. 2.2). Thus, sickle cell disease did not distinguish between the slave and the wealthy land-owner, and it does not distinguish between those who are black and those who are white. The populations sickle cell disease does single out are those from the tropical and subtropical climates of the Old World.

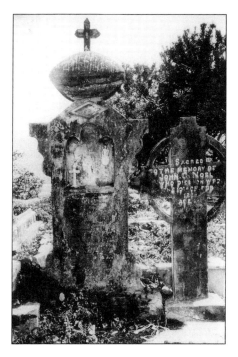

FIG. 2.2 The grave of Dr. Walter Clement Noel in the Catholic Cemetery of Sauters, Grenada, West Indies. Photo courtesy of Dr. Graham Serjeant (Medical Research Council Laboratories [Jamaica], University of the West Indies, Kingston).

The Malarial Hypothesis

Why the Old World and why the tropics? Why should this disease be so common in people of African descent? And why somewhat less common in people from other Old World tropical areas? Answers to these questions began to materialize in the 1940s, when E. A. Beet, a British colonial medical officer stationed in Northern Rhodesia (now Zimbabwe), observed that blood from malaria patients who had sickle cell trait (one Hb S gene and one Hb A gene, as discussed in Chapter 1) had fewer malarial parasites than blood from patients without the trait. (Parasites are living things that live in or on other living things and obtain nourishment from them.) Following this observation, a physician in Zaire reported that there were fewer cases of severe malaria (where parasites had infected the brain) among people with sickle cell trait than among those without it. In 1954, Anthony C. Allison, building on such observations, hypothesized that sickle cell trait offered protection against malaria. People with the trait, he suggested, did not succumb to malaria as often as people without it, and when they did, their disease was less severe.

In the following years, a body of information in support of Allison's hypothesis began to collect, but so did some evidence against it. The evidence against it showed no difference in the concentration of blood-borne malarial parasites in people with sickle cell trait and in those without it. When the studies were restricted to young people, however, the hypothesis held: sickle cell trait offered protection against malaria to *children*. Most adults who were stricken with malaria were able to develop *antibodies* (chemicals produced by the immune system that attack foreign material) to the parasite, and although their immunity was only partial, it helped them survive. For them, sickle cell trait offered little additional advantage. Youngsters, however, are not able to produce antibodies to the malarial parasite until their immune systems mature. Thus, it was the pre-immune malarial patients whose survival was protected by sickle cell trait. For them, too, protection was only partial, but they, too, survived. (Infants are not included in the group protected by sickle cell trait; antibodies produced by the mother's immune system circulate in the blood of the newborn, protecting them for a few months after birth.)

Several studies of malaria epidemics have indeed revealed a higher survival rate for sickle cell trait individuals than for those who lack Hb S. The malarial hypothesis is supported by those studies as well as by these other lines of evidence:

Geographic distribution. Malaria and sickle cell disease share the same geographic distribution. Figure 2.3 illustrates the distribution of the Hb S gene. These are the tropical and semi-tropical regions of Africa, the Arabian peninsula, India, and the Mediterranean Basin, the same regions where malaria is common. The malaria-sickle cell association also holds up within national boundaries. In Togo, for example, malaria is common in the lowlands but not in the mountains, and sickle cell genes, too, are common in the lowlands but not in the mountains. And although sickle cell genes are also found where malaria is not common, they did not originate there; they got there by migration. Although malaria epidemics have also occurred in the New World, none was recorded before the arrival of Columbus. The first severe epidemics were noted in 1493.

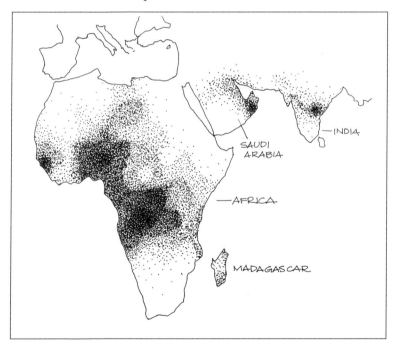

FIG. 2.3 The distribution of the sickle cell gene

Malaria probably originated in East Africa, around Ethiopia, and its carrier, the *Anopheles* mosquito, lived there long before people ever arrived on the scene. When people did arrive, they supplied the ingredient that enabled the malarial parasite to take up residence there—human flesh and blood. And when humans migrated, the parasite migrated, too. Eventually, it spread throughout the Old World tropics. That the geographic distribution of sickle cell trait corresponds to the geographic distribution of malaria supports an antimalarial role for sickle cell trait.

Gene frequency. The frequency of the sickle cell gene is too high in certain populations to be the result of mutation alone. Mutations occur all the time, but at low rates. Any one mutation is a rare event. Mutations that are disadvantageous are found at very low frequencies. This is because the people who carry them generally have few or no children. Mutations that are neutral—neither helpful nor harmful—are inherited along with the rest of the genome, and their frequency in the population usually does not increase very much. When a mutation is advantageous, however, people with the mutation have more children than people without it, and the frequency of that gene increases, sometimes rapidly. Since the frequency of the sickle cell gene is so high in certain populations, it must confer a selective advantage to that population: people with the gene have more children than people without the gene. The elevated frequency of the sickle cell gene among the populations exposed to malaria supports the malarial hypothesis.

"Transgenic" mice. One of the techniques developed by molecular biologists is the transplantation of genes from one species into individuals of another species. The recipient of the foreign gene is called *transgenic.* In an attempt to make an animal model for the study of sickle cell disease, human Hb S genes have been transplanted into mice. When two groups of

mice identical in every way, except that one group carried a single human Hb S gene, were both infected with malarial parasites, those with the Hb S gene had a less severe form of sickle cell disease. This supports the hypothesis that sickle cell hemoglobin confers protection against malaria.

Natural Selection

Everyone recognizes that life forms are different in different environments. Mosses live where it is wet, cactus plants live where it is dry. Dark-skinned people live where the sun's rays are strong and plentiful (pigmented skin protects against the harmful effects of the sun). Light-skinned people live where there is a poor supply of sunshine (the sun's radiation converts chemicals in the skin to vitamin D, and if dark skin pigments were to block out the sun in northern areas, growing children would suffer from a vitamin D deficiency). All living things adapt to the environments they live in. They do so by both chance mutations and chance recombinations of genes (see Chapter 1). Groups that do not adapt eventually die out. This process was discovered by Charles Darwin, who named it *natural selection,* or *survival of the fittest.*[8] The prevalence of Hb S genes in populations where malaria is endemic is a good example of natural selection.

Things that make an area particularly prone to malaria are stagnant pools of warm water where mosquitoes can breed (preferably all year long) and a malnourished population that lacks immunity to the disease. Malaria is a devastating and ancient disease. The enlarged spleens observed in three thousand-year-old mummies are believed to have been due to malaria. Malaria is mentioned in a papyrus from 1570 B.C.E.and was described in some detail by Hippocrates in the 5th century B.C.E. Hippocrates noted that there was a connection between marsh water and large, stiff spleens and death. Thus, the connection

between malaria and swampy, marshy areas has long been recognized. Indeed, the name of the disease comes from the Italian *mal aria*, evil air.

Although rainfall is often the cause of the stagnant water
where the *Anopheles* mosquito breeds, drought can also be. In
India, for example, heavy rains following the seasonal mon-
soons keep the rivers running. Periodically, however, the mon-
soons do not come and the rains do not fall. Rivers are then
converted into stagnant pools where mosquitoes thrive. This
sequence of events brought a major epidemic to Ceylon (now
Sri Lanka) in 1934.

Malaria is the most prevalent infectious disease in the world
today. About one billion people have malaria, and epidemics
take millions of lives each year in Africa alone. The symptoms
of malaria include periodic chills and fever (105° F), headache,
muscle pain, enlarged spleen, and anemia. Natural selection
against malaria was a welcome development.

Natural selection is a genetic process. Like heredity, it is a
matter of luck. The Hb S mutation did not develop for the purpose of protecting people against malaria—it developed by
chance. The first people who happened by chance to be carrying the Hb S gene when malaria struck were the lucky ones because more of them survived. More of their children survived,
too, and more of their children's children survived. Eventually,
so many of the survivors in malaria-infested areas carried the
Hb S gene that they began to marry one another. That is when
the less fortunate aspect of the protection came into play:
whenever two people carrying sickle cell trait married, one-
quarter of their children were born with sickle cell disease (see
Chapter 1).

In the original setting, most children with sickle cell disease
died during their first few years of life. When malaria came
around, however, most "normal" children (children who carried only Hb A genes) also died in their first few years of life. A
large proportion of children with sickle cell trait (one Hb S

gene and one Hb A gene), however, survived. This continued generation after generation, naturally selecting the Hb S-carrying population by granting life more often to those who—by chance—carried one Hb S gene and one Hb A gene.

We do not know when the life-saving Hb S mutation originated, but it was probably present when societies became agricultural, which was about two to three thousand years ago in Africa and about four thousand years ago in India. When social groups make the historic transition from food-gathering to food-producing economies, they change the ecology as well. First, they clear land for planting, exposing its waters to sunlight. This warmed water provides the kind of breeding grounds the *Anopheles* mosquito loves. Second, they form settlements, and this makes it easier for mosquitoes to thrive and to spread disease. Humans work the land. Mosquitoes work the humans. Malaria flourishes.

Since malaria was such a ravaging disease and sickle cell hemoglobin such an effective protection against it, it would not be surprising if natural selection for sickle cell mutations arose more than once. Modern techniques of genetic analysis have been used to explore this important evolutionary question.[9] One technique takes advantage of the fact that genes close together on the same chromosome are usually inherited together. Thus, relatives with sickle cell hemoglobin share not only the Hb S gene, but also the hemoglobin gene's neighboring genes. Such a cluster of DNA is called a *haplotype*. Members of the same tribe and people whose Hb S genes descend from the same ancestors will possess the same haplotype. By examining haplotypes, we can learn something about the migration and evolution of populations. In addition, we can learn whether the course of sickle cell disease is influenced by the haplotype.

A molecular technique applied to the study of sickle cell haplotypes uses *recognition-site enzymes*. Such enzymes recognize a specific bit of DNA called a "marker." Whenever a recognition-site enzyme finds its marker, it cuts through the

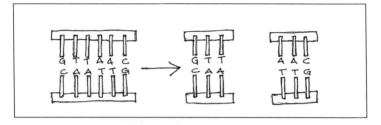

FIG. 2.4 The recognition sequence C-T-T-A-A-C being cut by a recognition-site enzyme

1) A–A–C 〰〰〰 Hb– S 〰〰〰 C–T–T

2) A–A –C 〰〰〰 Hb– S 〰〰〰〰〰 C–T–T

FIG. 2.5 Two different samples of DNA after treatment with recognition-site enzymes. The DNA lengths to the right of the Hb S genes are different, indicating that the two patients have different genetic backgrounds, or haplotypes. Thus, the patients are not closely related even though their Hb S genes are the same.

DNA at that site, chopping the molecule into smaller pieces (fig. 2.4). Thus, researchers can take a sample of tissue from patients with sickle cell disease, extract its DNA, and isolate the portion carrying the sickle cell gene. Then, using recognition-site enzymes, they cut this portion up and see what it is like. If the cut-up pieces from different patients are the same, then their haplotypes are the same, and they have likely descended from the same ancestors (fig. 2.5).

Recognition-site enzyme techniques have been used to study the evolution of sickle cell disease among various African populations. These studies revealed that the Hb S gene was present in at least four different haplotypes. This suggests that the Hb S gene arose among four different groups of people. And that suggests that there were at least four independent Hb S mutations, one associated with each of the four different haplotypes. Moreover, the groups carrying these haplotypes were geographically separated. That is, in each of four geographic areas, the sickle cell gene was associated almost exclusively with one particular haplotype. This is convincing evidence for four centers of origin for sickle cell disease in Africa. The four places in Africa where sickle cell mutations evidently originated are Central West Africa (the *Benin* haplotype), Atlantic West Africa around the Congo and Zaire (the *Senegal* haplotype), equatorial eastern and southern Africa (the *Bantu* haplotype), and central Cameroon (the *Cameroon* haplotype). A fifth mutation originated in either central India or eastern Saudi Arabia (the *Arab-Indian* haplotype) and spread from one to the other.

After their early appearances, sickle cell genes became more common as the populations that carried them grew by natural selection. Then, as people carrying the genes migrated, the genes spread to other populations. When sickle cell genes reached other areas of malarial infestation, they conferred an advantage and therefore expanded more.

Over the centuries, the independent Hb S mutations spread from their centers of origin to North Africa, the Middle East, southern Europe (around the Mediterranean), India, and the New World. They reached these areas when their carriers became involved in trade, warfare, migration, piracy, or slavery. Only the Cameroon haplotype did not migrate very much; except for a few cases found in adjacent Nigeria and America, and a few more scattered elsewhere, this haplotype remained within the tribe of its origin (the Etons).

Genetic studies of patients with sickle cell disease in North Africa, including Morocco, Algeria, Egypt, and Tunisia, show their Hb S genes to be linked to the Benin haplotype. Evidence suggests that during the Stone Age, the carriers of these genes traveled from Central West Africa across the then-fertile Sahara to the north. The presence of malaria among agricultural settlements there favored the Hb S gene. Later, as the Sahara began to dry up, there was a surge of migration away from the desert in all directions, spreading the gene further.

The major haplotype found in the Middle East among Syrians, Israeli Jews, and western Saudi Arabians is also Benin, and it probably got there from North Africa. Some evidence suggests that Israeli Arabs carry the Benin haplotype, too. In contrast to western Saudi Arabians, among whom the Benin haplotype is a reflection of the Arab slave trade, the eastern Saudi Arabians, like the Indians, carry the Arab-Indian haplotype. In India, the sickle cell gene is found primarily in isolated white tribal communities, but not in the majority population. The disease associated with the Arab-Indian haplotype is quite mild. This mildness is due to other hemoglobin mutations that modify the effect of Hb S (see Chapter 3). Some of the Arab-Indian haplotype may also exist in Iran.

The Benin haplotype is the only one found among sickle cell patients in all but one (Portugal) of the Mediterranean countries of Europe, including Spain, Sicily, Albania, Greece, and Turkey. The movement of these Central West African genes has been attributed to centuries of slave trading, invasions, and occupations by Muslims, Saracens, Arabs, Venetians, Ottomans, and Franks. In Portugal, however, the sickle cell genes that have been analyzed are linked primarily to the Bantu and Senegal haplotypes. This finding fits in with that country's exploitation of Africa; Portugal established control in the Bantu-inhabited areas of Angola and Mozambique (where they obtained slaves for their Brazilian colonies) and in Atlantic West Africa, near Senegal (then Portuguese Guinea, where they obtained slaves for their nearby Cape Verde Islands settlements).[10]

In the Americas, although some Hb S genes arrived with immigrants from the Mediterranean area, most came in the holds of slave ships. It is estimated that almost ten million Africans were shipped to the Americas during the seventeenth to nineteenth centuries. Today, genetic analysis of sickle cell patients reflects the geographic origins of those abducted ancestors. Genetic studies as well as historical records indicate that different sections of the New World selected their slaves from different parts of the Old.

Jamaica, for example, was the slave import hub for the British. Recent genetic analysis of a sickle cell disease population in Jamaica showed 72 percent to have the Benin haplotype, 17 percent to have the Bantu haplotype, and 10 percent to have the Senegal haplotype. Since slave ship records show that 747,500 slaves were brought to Jamaica from 1655 to 1807, the haplotype analyses suggest that 538,200 slaves came from Central West Africa, 127,075 came from Bantu Africa, and 74,750 came from Atlantic West Africa. These numbers correspond closely with actual slave trade records, which demonstrates the analytical power of haplotype studies; DNA is history's scrapbook.

Haplotype analysis of a Baltimore sickle cell patient population indicates that, again, the largest proportion, 62 percent, of their antecedents came from Central West Africa (Benin haplotype), whereas 18 percent came from Bantu Africa and 15 percent came from Atlantic West Africa. Again, these percentages agree with old slave records; in this case, the records were of the eighteenth century British Virginia slave trade. South Carolina slave trade records reveal different practices. In contrast to Virginia, South Carolina imported most of its slaves from Atlantic West Africa (they carried the Senegal haplotype), not from Central West Africa. From 1733 to 1807, 43 percent of South Carolina's slave imports were from Atlantic West Africa, 40 percent were from Bantu Africa, and only 17 percent were from Central West Africa. This ratio is echoed by today's black population in the United States' South. And the DNA of black Americans reflects this ancestry.

In the New York area, the second largest group of sickle cell disease patients are of Sicilian ancestry. Dr. Ronald Nagel of the

Albert Einstein College of Medicine in New York explains that about twelve hundred years ago, Arabs carrying the sickle cell trait invaded Sicily. Since malaria was a serious problem there, the gene was a welcome introduction, and it thrived. Today, 13 percent of the people in the Sicilian city of Butera carry the sickle cell gene. Dr. Nagel recounts why: The area around Butera and Gela has been the preferred landing site of all the invaders of Sicily. That's where the Arabs landed. The reason is that there is a very small rise in the terrain, and then you can go to Palermo and to Catania and dominate Sicily. General Patton did the same thing in World War II. He landed in Gela, just as the Arabs had done centuries before. And you can still see the pillboxes the Germans set up there because they suspected that this might be one of the Allied Forces' landing sites. According to the people in Butera, the Arabs settled in Butera and set up a Sudanese detachment. This brought a significant influx of sickle cell genes that expanded even more with malaria.[11]

When a disease as devastating as malaria threatens the populations of extensive geographic areas, it is not surprising that an adaptation to it—sickle cell hemoglobin—developed independently at least five times. It would also not be surprising if sickle cell hemoglobin was not the only adaptation to malaria to have evolved. Other hemoglobin adaptations have, in fact, evolved in malaria-infested areas. Among these are hemoglobin C, a mutant hemoglobin, and the thalassemias, a group of conditions that affect the amount of hemoglobin produced, rather than the type. Some people with sickle cell genes also have genes for these.

About 1 in 835 African Americans is born with both a Hb S gene and a Hb C gene. These people have a milder form of sickle cell disease than people with two Hb S genes (see Chapter 3). About 1 in 1,667 African Americans is born with a Hb S gene and a beta thalassemia gene. Hb S-beta thalassemia disease is variable; it ranges from being indistinguishable from ordinary sickle cell disease to being almost symptom-free, depending on the nature of the thalassemia mutation.

The Gene Persists

It should now be clear why the sickle cell gene expanded in tropical areas hospitable to malaria. But this does not explain why the gene (and therefore the disease) persists in descendants who no longer live with malaria. As you might have guessed, the Hb S gene has become less common among American blacks than it was among their African forebears. But genes do not disappear merely because they no longer serve a useful purpose. As a rule, genes remain stable in a population unless something causes them to increase or to decrease in frequency (that's natural selection at work). Since the frequency of the sickle cell gene has decreased among American blacks, something must be causing this to happen. Two possibilities come to mind. First, Hb S genes could have become diluted through interracial matings. Second, there could have been natural selection against the Hb S gene: when there is no malaria to favor the Hb S gene and ill health takes its toll among people carrying two copies of the Hb S gene, fewer children carrying the Hb S gene are born.

We can search for evidence in support of the two possibilities, realizing that it also may be that both of them are operative. One genetic study indicates that about 20 percent of blood group genes (we mean here the ABO blood groups) in African Americans are of white origin. This indicates that the first possibility holds: blacks and whites have become racially mixed in America, and black genes are therefore diluted with white genes. This is no surprise, especially since black women slaves were commonly raped by their white owners. A study of hemoglobin genes in African Americans, however, indicates an even higher percentage of nonblack representation; that is, *more* than 20 percent of the hemoglobin genes of black-Americans are of white origin. This selective decrease of black hemoglobin genes suggests that the second possibility also holds: blacks who carry sickle cell genes have had fewer children than blacks who do not. This is no surprise either, since black people with two Hb S genes rarely used to survive to reproductive age. Thus, racial mixing and natural selection both seem to have played a role in reducing the frequency of the sickle cell gene in black Americans.

Another factor, however, could halt the gradual decrease of sickle cell genes that is occurring in America. So much has been learned about sickle cell disease, and patient care has so improved in recent years, that about 90 percent of sickle cell disease patients now reach reproductive age. This means that natural selection against sickle cell disease may no longer reduce the number of sickle cell genes in the African-American population. On the other hand, modern medicine and birth control techniques can now help parents who do not want to bring a sickle cell child into the world (see Chapter 6), and "unnatural" selection against sickle cell disease could take over where natural selection leaves off.

3. Inside the Red Blood Cell

In 1773, William Hewson, the English physician who became the "father of hematology" (and the son-in-law of Benjamin Franklin's landlady in England), wrote that the "red particles of the blood...must be of great use" because they appear "so generously" among all the different animals.[12] Hewson's logic was certainly sound, but evidence in support of it was not forthcoming for almost a century. In the 1860s, a German scientist, Felix Hoppe-Seyler, showed that the red material inside the red blood cell could take up and release oxygen. He showed that the material was a two-part, iron-containing protein, which he named "hemoglobin." The two parts of hemoglobin are *heme*, the iron-holding unit, and *globin*, the surrounding protein. The heme is the part that combines with oxygen, picking it up in the lungs and releasing it in tissues where there is less oxygen. One heme unit attaches to four protein chains (two alpha chains and two beta chains) in a hemoglobin molecule, so one hemoglobin molecule carries four oxygen molecules.

Humans need oxygen to process their food. A person who consumes 2000 calories in a day needs about 400 liters (95 gallons) of oxygen, or about one cup of oxygen per minute, to process it. One cup of oxygen contains roughly about 6,500,000,000,000,000,000,000 oxygen molecules. Supplying this is a big-time job. Picking up oxygen where it is plentiful (in the lungs) and releasing it where it is lacking is one part of the job; Hb S does that part well—just as well as Hb A does. Carrying the oxygen through blood vessels is another part of the job, and that is the part that Hb S often sabotages.

The red cell is primarily a sack of hemoglobin. Transporting hemoglobin is almost the only thing the red blood cell does. Unlike other cells of the body, the red cell does not reproduce—it is made by *stem cells* in the bone marrow—and it does not even contain a nucleus. Ninety percent of the weight

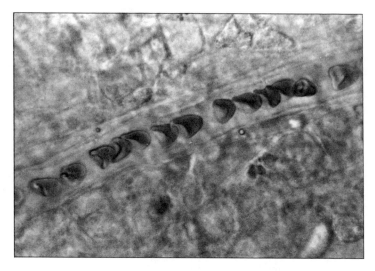

FIG. 3.1 Red blood cells flowing through a small blood vessel. Photo courtesy of Dr. P.-I. Brånemark (Institute of Applied Biotechnology, Gothenburg, Sweden) and Dr. R. Skalak (University of California, San Diego).

of a red blood cell is hemoglobin, and each cell contains about 265,000,000 hemoglobin molecules. Red cells containing normal hemoglobin, and red cells containing sickle cell hemoglobin under nonsickling conditions, are shaped like flattened discs with a pinched center (frontispiece), and they are flexible; they can change their shape as their job requires. As they squeeze through small blood vessels, normal red cells assume the shape of a bullet (fig. 3.1). Sickle cells cannot do this, however, and the problem lies with Hb S.

Polymers

Hemoglobin solutions can be extracted from red blood cells and examined in the laboratory. This has been done with Hb A and Hb S in experiments that studied the effect of different oxygen concentrations. When oxygen was plentiful in these experiments, solutions of Hb A and Hb S behaved pretty much the same way. When oxygen was lacking, however, the two kinds of hemoglobin solutions behaved very differently. The Hb A molecules remained in a liquid solution. The Hb S molecules, however, came out of solution. They grew thicker and then half-solid (like gelatin), and rigid, crystal-like solids formed. When oxygen was added back, the Hb S dissolved and the solution became liquid again. What are these solids that form in Hb S solutions when the oxygen supply is low? These are neighboring Hb S molecules that come together and stick to each other. The process is called *polymerization*, and the large, compound molecule formed is called a *polymer*. Hb S polymerization forms rigid, rope-like chains that resemble bunches of wire.

Inside the red blood cell, hemoglobin molecules behave the same way they did in the experiment described above. As oxygen becomes depleted, the Hb A solution remains liquid. The Hb S solution, however, becomes thicker, and then the Hb S molecules come together and polymerize. Just as they do in a laboratory dish, the polymers form rigid, rope-like chains that resemble bunches of wire. These "wires" distort the shape of the red cell, damaging it as well. Because the distorted cells often resemble a sickle (a curved farming implement, the one that crosses with a hammer on the flag of the former Soviet Union), they are called "sickle cells" (frontispiece). When oxygen is returned to the cell, the Hb S redissolves. Under low oxygen conditions, then, a red blood cell containing Hb A is like a filled water balloon at room temperature. It can easily be squeezed and bent. A red blood cell containing Hb S, on the other hand, is like a water balloon that has spent a few hours in the freezer. It is not flexible, it cannot be bent, and there is no way it can be squeezed through a tube that is narrower than the balloon itself.

The Hb S polymer has been extensively studied. It appears to be made up of seven double cords of Hb S twisted together like a rope. The rope is formed in stages. First, nearby Hb S molecules come together and form many small cords. These contain perhaps two to five Hb S molecules each. Then, at an unknown signal, polymers begin a rapid growth phase. Free Hb S molecules attach to the outsides of the existing cords, causing them to grow rapidly into long rods that line up in parallel. It is these rods that take away the red cell's flexibility (like ice in the water balloon). The longer the hemoglobin is without oxygen, the longer the rods grow. Thus, when red blood cells travel through the small vessels in tissues with low oxygen content, it is important for them to get out quickly, before the hemoglobin polymerizes. When polymers form and when sickling occurs, the red cells cannot assume their bullet shape and shoot through the vessels. Moreover, the variety of shapes they do assume are not conducive to flow. To make matters worse, the problem of having an unstreamlined shape is often compounded by hairlike projections or spikes that extend out from the cell, making the cells sticky.

As was mentioned before, if the polymer becomes exposed to oxygen it can melt back to individual Hb S molecules again. The polymers in the hairlike membrane projections also dissolve and flow back into the body of the cell. If the polymer dissolves in *reversibly sickled cells*, they will get back their normal shape and resume red cell function. Even so, they have been damaged. After repeated sickling episodes, or long ones, cells become *irreversibly sickled*. Irreversibly sickled cells are permanently deformed; they do not resume normal shape even when the polymers within them are redissolved. Thus, Hb S polymers permanently damage the red cell membrane, shortening the lifespan of the cell. Irreversibly sickled cells are destroyed.

Several factors influence Hb S polymerization. These include the amount of oxygen present, the concentration of Hb S, and the kind and amount of other hemoglobins in the cell. The amount of oxygen present is of primary importance. This was discovered in 1927, when E. Vernon Hahn, a young surgeon in Indianapolis, happened to notice that many sickled cells in a patient's blood sample were sitting at the bottom of the collection tube. When he shook the tube, the sickled cells seemed to disappear. Since the concentration of oxygen is lowest at the bottom of a test tube, and since shaking the tube mixes fresh oxygen into it, Hahn reasoned that oxygen had something to do with sickling. That was good thinking. He and an intern conducted experiments to test this idea. They suspended some blood in a glass chamber positioned under a microscope lens and observed it while they passed different gas mixtures through the chamber. Their observations confirmed that oxygen deficiency causes sickling, and they went on to define the oxygen level that makes it happen. They also took the hemoglobin out of some cells and studied the emptied cells under low oxygen conditions. Because these red cell "ghosts" did not sickle, they concluded that hemoglobin is the molecule that is responsible for sickling in sickle cell disease, and that sickling is a response to low oxygen levels. When low oxygen levels in body tissues cause red blood cells to sickle, the situation grows worse. Flow slows down. Blood backs up. The stagnant blood loses more oxygen, causing even more sickling.

Hemoglobin concentration is another factor that influences sickling. In a concentrated solution, molecules are closer together. The closer molecules are, the more likely they are to come into contact with each other. When Hb S molecules come into contact with one another, they polymerize to form the rigid rods that cause the cells to sickle. One of the reasons that people with sickle cell disease are encouraged to drink large amounts of fluids (Chapter 5) is that fluids cause the red blood cell to absorb more water, and water dilutes the hemoglobin.

Sickling is greatly influenced by the presence of other hemoglobins. The kind as well as the amount matters. In sickle cell trait, where some of the hemoglobin in the cell is Hb S and the rest is Hb A, Hb S does not usually polymerize. There are two reasons for this. First, the more Hb A there is, the less Hb S there is, so less Hb S is available for polymer formation. Second, Hb A does not readily enter into polymers. Hb C also does not readily polymerize, but people with one gene for Hb C and one for Hb S still have sickle cell disease. This is because such people produce a greater proportion of Hb S than do people with sickle cell trait, and also because the hemoglobin in their cells is more concentrated; both of these factors make the Hb S more likely to polymerize. The sickle cell disease symptoms in people with one Hb C and one Hb S gene are usually milder than they are in people with two Hb S genes (Chapter 4).

Fetal hemoglobin (Hb F) decreases sickling in the same two ways as Hb A, but its globin chains do not enter polymers at all. Thus, it inhibits polymerization even more than Hb A, and infants with sickle cell disease do not show any disease symptoms as long as they have a large number of red cells with a lot of Hb F in them (Chapter 4). People with sickle cell disease whose chromosomes reveal the Arab-Indian haplotype (Chapter 2) generally produce high levels of Hb F. The mild form of disease usually found with this haplotype is believed related to those high Hb F levels. Also, there are some sickle cell people with a mutation that causes them to make large amounts of Hb F as adults, and these people, too, generally have a mild form of sickle cell disease.

Although several studies have reported that symptoms are more likely to occur when the weather turns colder or when individual patients are subject to cold, sickling itself is not related to temperature. People with sickle cell disease are advised to protect themselves against the cold (Chapter 5), but the reason that problems sometimes arise when temperatures drop is not understood.

Parasites

Now that we have examined the role of Hb S in sickle cell disease, let's take a look at its role in malaria. The malarial parasite has a complex and fascinating life cycle that requires two hosts—the human and the female *Anopheles* mosquito. (The female needs to eat blood to produce fertile eggs; the male is a vegetarian.) When an infected female *Anopheles* mosquito bites a person, it injects some parasites into that person's blood stream. After a while, the parasites enter the red blood cells, eat everything in them, and divide into many smaller parasites. The infected red blood cells then break open, spilling the parasites and their products into the blood stream. (This is when chills, fever, and sweating occur.) The released parasites then invade fresh red blood cells and start a new cycle. After many such cycles, the parasites develop into a form that does not rupture the host red blood cell but remains inside. If this red blood cell is eaten by a female *Anopheles* mosquito, the parasites live in the mosquito—that's where they have their sex life—until they are ready to infect a human again. This they do when their mosquito hostess finds a new human to dine upon.

If the next person has sickle cell trait, however, the parasites have a problem. They are not able to infect the red blood cells as easily, nor do they develop as successfully within them. Why this is so is not yet fully understood. Here are some possibilities:

1. The parasite inside the red cell produces acid. In the presence of acid, the Hb S has a tendency to polymerize, and this causes the cell to sickle. Since sickled cells are destroyed as the blood circulates through the spleen, the parasites are destroyed, too.

2. Malarial parasites do not live long under low oxygen conditions. Since the oxygen concentration is low in the spleen, and since infected red cells tend to get trapped in the spleen, they may be killed there.

3. Another thing that happens under low oxygen conditions is that potassium leaks out of Hb S-containing cells. The parasite needs high potassium levels to develop, so this may be the reason the parasite fails to thrive in red blood cells containing Hb S.

Regardless of the explanation, people with sickle cell trait have milder cases of malaria because they are host to fewer and weaker parasites.

4. Possible Effects of Sickle Cell Disease

People with sickle cell disease are living longer, fuller, and more comfortable lives than ever before. In 1973, the average lifespan of a person with sickle cell anemia was a little over 14 years. Now, it is 42 years for men and 48 years for women, and some live many years longer. The average life span for people with sickle cell-hemoglobin C disease is 60 years for men and 68 for women. These increased lifespans follow from an increased understanding of the biology of the disease, which has led to better medical care and fulfillment of the nutritional and educational needs of the sickle cell patient. Moreover, earlier diagnosis has meant that a program of life-prolonging care, with emphasis on the prevention of problems, could begin in the first few months of life, a time when so many used to succumb. It is not possible to tell in advance how much a person's life will be affected by sickle cell disease. The course of the disease is not the same for everyone, not even for everyone in the same family. It is not even the same for the same person at different times of life. The disease is severe for some individuals and quite mild for others. The reasons for this are not yet understood, although some of the things that influence the disease are recognized. These influences can be genetic or nongenetic.

Genetic factors that influence sickle cell disease include the production of other types of hemoglobin, haplotypes (Chapter 2), and the thalassemias. About 2 percent of African Americans carry a gene for Hb C. Hb C in combination with Hb S tends to produce a milder disease. Some people who make both Hb S and Hb C have so few symptoms that they do not even realize they have sickle cell disease. Their childhood growth is normal. They usually do not have symptoms in their first year of life and may not have them for many years. Most complications of the disease are rare. The more common complications involve the spleen, the eyes, and the chest.

The human fetus produces its own type of hemoglobin, Hb F. Some people carry a mutation that causes them to continue making Hb F after birth. These people do not suffer sickle cell disease symptoms even when 70 percent of their hemoglobin is Hb S. People with the Arab-Indian type of chromosome (Chapter 2) also produce high levels of Hb F, and they usually have mild forms of the disease. People with the Senegal haplotype, who often have mild disease, produce relatively high amounts of Hb F, and women produce more than men. In sickle cell patients in general, high Hb F levels are associated with a longer lifespan. The relationship between Hb F and disease severity is not simple, however, and mildness of symptoms is not always associated with elevated Hb F levels.

Thalassemia is more than one disease. Some thalassemia mutations reduce globin chain production by a small amount, some by a large amount, some completely. Alpha thalassemia reduces the number of alpha chains produced; beta thalassemia reduces the number of beta chains produced (normal ones). In either case, when the cell tries to make some ordinary hemoglobin molecules out of two alpha chains and two beta chains, it doesn't have the right supply of parts. The alpha thalassemias seem to lessen some of the symptoms of sickle cell disease and to make others worse. Different beta thalassemias have different effects. If the mutation blocks all production of normal beta chains, people with one beta thalassemia gene and one Hb S gene have the same symptoms as people with two Hb S genes. Other beta thalassemia mutations permit the production of some normal beta chains. People who carry one of these genes and one Hb S gene will make some Hb A and will therefore have a milder disease.

One nongenetic factor that is a major influence on the course of sickle cell disease is nutrition. Another is medical

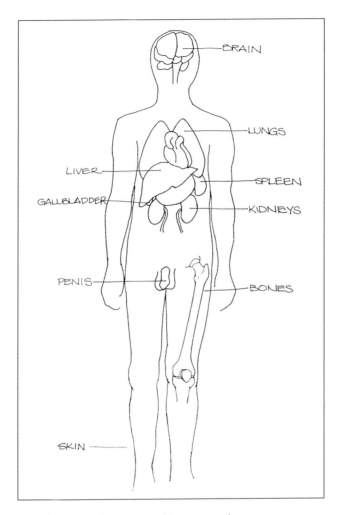

FIG. 4.1 The organs that cause problems most often

care. Proper nutrition plus good medical care, along with support from knowledgeable, caring family and friends, can do much to improve the course of the illness.

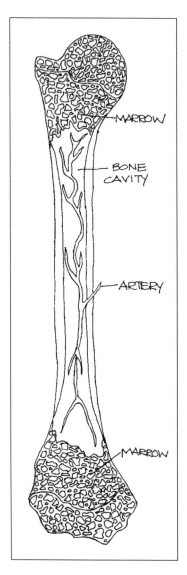

FIG. 4.2 Inside the upper arm bone, one of the places where blood cells are made

The Symptoms of Sickle Cell Disease

Sickle cell disease hurts—not always, and not necessarily often, but painful episodes are characteristic of the disease. Painful episodes may last a few days, which is usually the case, or they may last for weeks. They range in intensity from annoying to excruciating. Other problems also commonly beset people with sickle cell disease. These include increased vulnerability to infection, anemia, organ damage, and a tendency to form gallstones. All of these problems follow from the single original problem in sickle cell disease: abnormal hemoglobin. Emotional problems can be expected to follow the physical ones.

Painful episodes

Most of the pain of sickle cell disease occurs when abnormal blood cells block small blood vessels. When the vessels are blocked, blood cannot flow through them and deliver oxygen to the parts of the body supplied by those vessels. When body parts are deprived of oxygen, they release chemicals that cause pain; if blood flow is not restored soon, tissue damage follows. Where tissue is damaged the area becomes *inflamed* (filled with special cells that dispose of dead tissue), and this, too, becomes a source of pain. Fever often accompanies episodes of pain. Since any of the small blood vessels may become blocked at any time in sickle cell disease, pain and tissue damage can occur anywhere in the body, and it is impossible to predict when and where it will happen next.

The parts of the body in which painful episodes are most common are the bones, chest, and abdomen (fig. 4.1). The intensity and duration of the pain, which are variable, guide its treatment. For mild to intermediate pain, simple medication such as acetaminophen or codeine may provide relief, and water should be drunk. For intense and enduring pain, the physician may give stronger pain-killing drugs, such as morphine and *intravenous* (into the vein) fluids. Often, it is necessary to treat more than the pain, for pain is a symptom of underlying trouble. The special skills of a physician are required to determine the cause of the pain and to devise appropriate treatment.

Bones. Although skeletons are often used to symbolize death, the bones of a living person are very much alive. The job of bones, in addition to providing the body with a movable structural and protective support, is to manufacture blood cells. This is done by *marrow*, a soft, netlike mass of tissue found inside certain bones (fig. 4.2). The marrow is particularly active in people with sickle cell disease because defective red blood cells are regularly being destroyed elsewhere in the body and must be replaced.

Like all other living tissues, bones need a constant blood supply. Circulation in the bone, however, faces obstacles. Blood must travel through many tiny openings, or *sinusoids*, in sponge-like parts of bone. In sickle cell disease, the inflexible and sickled blood cells often get trapped in sinusoids. This blocks the circulation, causing bone and joint pain, one of the most frequent problems in the disease. The pain generally lasts several days. In the very young, blocked blood flow in the bones of the hands and feet causes local swelling accompanied by pain and fever. This is called *hand-foot syndrome*. (A *syndrome* is a collection of symptoms that together are typical of a specific condition.) Since hand-foot syndrome is often the first symptom of the disease a child may display, its appearance is frequently the way parents learn that their child has the disease. Hand-foot syndrome usually lasts only about a week, even without medical treatment, but it can recur.

The location of bone pain usually changes as people grow. Older children often suffer episodes of pain in the bones of their arms and legs, and this may be accompanied by swelling and fever. The hip and shoulder joints are common sites of pain in the adolescent and adult. The hip joint, which bears a good deal of weight in routine day-to-day activities, can suffer serious damage if it is not cared for (by not walking, for example) during episodes of pain. Back pain, too, is common, whereas facial bone pain is not.

Chest. It is in the lungs that the red blood cells obtain the oxygen that they deliver to every cell in the body (and where they also get rid of waste carbon dioxide). The oxygen enters the lungs along with the fresh air we inhale as our chests expand. The chests of patients with sickle cell disease, however, are often narrower than normal, and the heart is often larger, both of which leave the lungs less space to work in. The less the lungs are able to expand, the less is the amount of oxygen that can be inhaled. Moreover, the volume of blood that passes through the lungs of sickle cell patients is larger than it is in healthy individuals, so more lung work is required. Thus, when a sickle cell person's lungs undergo blood vessel blockage or become infected, the situation is especially dangerous. Patients may be stricken with severe chest pain, fever, coughing, and difficulty in breathing; this is termed *acute chest syndrome*. There can also be accompanying bone pain. Since lung involvement can spread and even be fatal if appropriate treatment is not given, patients with acute chest syndrome should be taken to the hospital for care. Repeated incidents of acute chest syndrome can lead to chronic lung disease.

Abdomen. Blockage of blood vessels serving the abdominal region gives rise to abdominal pain that generally persists four or five days. Two vulnerable organs are the liver and the spleen. The liver is a large organ (even larger in people with sickle cell disease) in the upper right side of the abdominal cavity. It plays vital roles in digestion, excretion (ridding the body of waste material), energy metabolism (getting the energy from food calories), the removal of toxic products from the blood, and blood cell storage. Blood cells often become trapped in the liver in sickle cell disease, and the organ builds up pigment deposits, injuries, and scarring. When the liver is affected, patients feel pain in the right side of the abdomen and they are likely to have yellow in the whites of their eyes (*jaundice*), and fever. The source of the yellow color is *bilirubin*, a hemoglobin waste product that is removed from the blood plasma by the liver. Jaundice occurs when there is too much bilirubin around for the liver to process or when there is liver damage. Another way that the liver may be injured follows not from the disease but from its treatment. Blood transfusions, a frequent therapy for certain sickle cell disease symptoms, occasionally introduce a virus that causes *hepatitis*, a liver disease.

The spleen, situated in the upper left side of the abdominal cavity, serves as a blood reservoir: it stores blood when circulation is decreased (such as when the body is at rest) and it releases blood when circulation is increased (as when the body is doing exercise or bleeding). Normally, blood undergoes cleaning as it travels through the spleen. Old, damaged, and abnormal blood cells are destroyed there. If you are healthy, about 200 million of your old blood cells will be destroyed (and an equal amount of new ones made) in the time it takes you to read this page. The hemoglobin from those destroyed cells is converted to bilirubin in the spleen and excreted by the liver; the leftover cellular material is taken up by *phagocytes* (cells that devour and destroy particulate matter) in the spleen. These phagocytes also remove bacteria and other foreign material from the blood. Additionally, the spleen is an important antibody-producing organ of the immune system. Thus, the spleen combats infections in at least two different ways—by engulfing bacteria and by producing chemicals that attack foreign material. People with damaged spleens are prone to infection, especially when they are young.

Blood traveling through the spleen must work its way through an intricate network of finely branched vessels and squeeze through numerous tiny sinusoids. Since the red blood cells in sickle cell disease are not very flexible, they very often get stuck in the spleen. The organ becomes swollen and does not work as well. This commonly begins in very early childhood, and the organ progressively loses its ability to function. Over the years, with repeated damage and scarring, it gradually gets smaller and smaller. Sometimes, however, the spleen becomes chronically enlarged. In *splenic sequestration*, the enlarged spleen traps a large portion of the body's red blood cells so that inadequate numbers circulate. In *acute splenic sequestration* crises, the entrapment of a major portion of the body's red blood cells causes acute, life-threatening anemia that must be treated by transfusion. *Splenectomy* (surgical removal of the spleen) is sometimes performed to prevent recurrence of the episode, but the decision to perform a splenectomy is an onerous one: when the spleen is removed, so is its immune function, and the patient becomes even more susceptible to infection.

It is often not easy to predict when a painful episode will occur, but some things that appear to bring them on are infections, too little fluid intake, cold weather, excessive physical stress, and emotional pain.

Vulnerability to infection

Many of the symptoms caused by lack of oxygen could also be due to infections by *microorganisms* (germs), and physicians are always watchful of that possibility so that they can treat the patient appropriately. Microorganisms are everywhere. They are in us, they are on us, they surround us. They can gain entry into our bodies in many ways and rarely miss an opportunity to do so. We may breathe microorganisms in, and that is how the common cold and tuberculosis are contracted. We can eat them or their toxins, and that is how we get food poisoning. They can enter cuts and wounds, and this is what happens in skin infections and gangrene. They may enter ordinary body openings, as they do in ear and bladder infections. They may gain entry directly into the blood stream through the use of contaminated injection needles, as happens with AIDS (acquired immune deficiency syndrome) and some forms of hepatitis, and they may be deposited into the blood by insects such as mosquitoes, which is how malaria is spread.

The spleen is a major barrier to infection. Since the spleen is damaged and sometimes destroyed or surgically removed in sickle cell patients, these patients are particularly vulnerable to infection. And the younger patients are when spleen damage occurs, the more dangerous their childhoods will be. Other components of the body's immune defense system also seem to be abnormal in sickle cell disease. Once infected, therefore, sickle cell patients are harder to treat than healthy individuals, and their well-being can be more seriously threatened. Thus, an aggressive program to ward off infections is considered essential in the care of sickle cell disease patients. Sickle cell children should be given immunizations to diphtheria, whooping cough, tetanus, polio, measles, mumps, rubella, Hemophilus b, Pneumococcus, and anything else that the physician or sickle cell center recommends. In addition, sickle cell children are routinely given *prophylactic* (preventive) *antibiotics* (drugs that kill microorganisms).

Certain microorganisms seem to feel particularly at home with sickle cell disease. Among these, *Streptococcus pneumoniae* is especially dangerous to very young children. As sickle cell patients get older, diseases caused by this microorganism become relatively rare. In the absence of antibiotic treatment, *S. pneumoniae* can multiply profusely in the blood stream, causing *septicemia* (blood poisoning), or in the spinal fluid, causing *meningitis* (inflammation of the membranes that enclose the brain and spinal cord). Entry into the blood stream can be by inhalation; entry into the spinal fluid usually starts with an ear infection. Pneumococcal septicemia causes high fever, convulsions, confusion, and coma, and is often fatal. Pneumococcal meningitis brings about similar symptoms, and infections can recur. As with septicemia, attacks may be fatal. When they are not, there may be lasting effects, such as paralysis, deafness, blindness, or mental retardation. Prompt, intravenous administration of penicillin will normally rescue the patient and prevent lasting damage.

Other microorganisms of concern are *Hemophilus influenzae*, *Salmonella*, and *Escherichia coli*. *H. influenzae* is the cause of nose, throat, and ear infections, pneumonia, and meningitis. *Salmonella* is a frequent cause of *osteomyelitis* (bone inflammation) in young people with sickle cell disease. Its symptoms include fever, nausea, vomiting, and pain at the site of inflammation; muscles adjacent to the affected bone may go into spasms.

E. coli is the most common microorganism found in human feces (solid waste discharged by the intestine), and the bulk of feces is mostly microorganisms. *E. coli* can gain entry to the body through the urinary tract opening and travel up to the bladder. Bladder infections are more frequent in females than in males because female bladders are closer to the body opening where the bacteria get in. Although most strains of *E. coli* do not cause disease, some may lead to septicemia and osteomyelitis.

The microorganisms named above are a special problem in sickle cell disease. Any infectious agent, however, will bring more trouble to sickle cell people, particularly young ones, than to the general population. Microorganisms are great opportunists; when they find their way into a person with a weakened defense system, they reproduce and reproduce and reproduce. Thus, all signs of infection must be acted upon promptly.

Anemia

Although infections seem to be most problematic to young people, *anemia* (insufficient hemoglobin) is a problem for all age groups. Anemia may be due to too few red blood cells or to too little hemoglobin within them. It is a chronic condition in sickle cell disease. When red blood cells become sickled, they (and their hemoglobin) are destroyed. Whereas the average life of a normal red blood cell is 120 days, the average life of a red blood cell in a patient with sickle cell disease is only 20 days. This means that red cell production must proceed at an accelerated rate to replace all those that are being destroyed. The bone marrow (the organ that makes hemoglobin and red blood cells) may not be able to keep up with demand. This is because the marrow is invariably damaged or functionally impaired due to blockage of the blood vessels that supply it. Thus, some level of chronic anemia is characteristic of sickle cell disease.

More acute forms of anemia may also develop. One cause can be nutritional deficiencies. Among the materials needed for red blood cell production is a vitamin called *folic acid*. Since red blood cells are in full-time production in sickle cell disease, large amounts of the vitamin are used. Folic acid is widely distributed in plants and animals, so deficiencies are unusual. Nevertheless, dietary supplements of folic acid are sometimes needed, especially in poorly nourished patients, during pregnancy, and during the rapid growth surges of infancy and childhood. *Iron deficiency*, too, can cause anemia, especially during pregnancy, and dietary iron supplements are sometimes recommended.

In addition to nutritional deficiency, acute splenic sequestration, which has already been described, can cause anemia. You will recall that in this dangerous situation, the spleen becomes greatly enlarged and sequesters a large portion of the body's red blood cells, leaving too few in the circulation to sustain life. This condition usually occurs in young children; older ones generally do not have enough working spleen left to sequester much blood. Immediate blood transfusion is essential to counter the anemia.

Hypersplenism is another cause of anemic episodes. In this unusual condition, the spleen gets larger during the course of the disease, instead of smaller. Even more than the usual number of red blood cells are destroyed by the enlarged spleen, and the life of the red blood cell is even shorter. This takes a heavy toll on the body, which must provide the energy and nutrients to meet the demands of perpetual red cell production. Hence, children with hypersplenism are usually smaller for their age than other sickle cell children (who are also small for their age), and enlarged abdomens reflect their enlarged spleens. The condition is treated by chronic blood transfusions or by splenectomy.

In *aplastic crisis*, the production of red blood cells stops completely. The crisis may begin with headache, fever, fatigue, or abdominal or limb pain. The anemia is severe and is usually treated with blood transfusions. After five to ten days, the bone marrow recovers and red cell production resumes. Aplastic crisis is caused by a virus (parvovirus B19) that usually infects the young. Children do not become infected a second time, however, showing that they develop parvovirus immunity.

Other infectious agents may contribute to anemia in a secondary way. They may slow down the production of red blood cells, they may hasten their destruction, or they may further the likelihood of blood vessel blockage. Blood vessel blockage due to sickle cell disease is common in the kidney, causing it to become increasingly damaged with age. Chronic *kidney disease* is another route to anemia, due perhaps to the accumulation in the blood of marrow-depressing toxins normally removed by the kidney, or to a reduction of the amount of *erythropoietin* produced. Erythropoietin, a hormone that tells the bone marrow to make new red blood cells, is made in the kidney, and if the kidney is damaged, less erythropoietin (and therefore a smaller number of red blood cells) is made. The kidneys are also responsible for filtering metabolic wastes out of the blood, forming urine, and retaining the proper salt balance in the body; these functions are essential to life.

Organ damage

Several organs particularly subject to damage and associated with pain have already been discussed; these were the bones and joints, lungs, liver, and spleen. The damaged kidney was mentioned as a link to anemia. Damaged kidneys also do not concentrate urine normally, and this leads to frequent urination and bed-wetting. But any and all organs may be damaged, either by chronic anemia or by blocked blood vessels, both of which are characteristic of sickle cell disease. Eyes can be damaged and vision affected to various degrees. Some hearing loss, due perhaps to inadequate blood flow to the inner ear, is not unusual. Skin lesions can occur either spontaneously (due to blockage of small, superficial vessels) or in response to injury. Ulcerations (chronic sores) on the lower part of the leg, usually near the ankles and sometimes as wide as seven inches, become common in adulthood, especially in men, and may take months or even years to heal. Until they do heal, they are an ever present source of infection. Even after healing, the scar tissue may break down and ulceration occur again.

The heart is enlarged (because of its greater work load) and does not respond as effectively as the normal heart to increased exercise. Nevertheless, this organ seems relatively resistant to sickle cell disease damage, and patients do not demonstrate the symptoms of cardiovascular disease prevalent in the general American population. In later life, however, congestive heart failure commonly develops. Like the spleen, the penis has a complex network of blood vessels that is particularly vulnerable to blockage in sickle cell disease. Blockage of the outflow vessels can cause *priapism* (a prolonged, painful erection), which may be accompanied by swelling and by added pain during urination. Priapism can occur in very young boys as well as in older males. It may be associated with sexual activity with or without a partner. In some cases, erection lasts for a few hours at most and may not be very painful, but it often recurs. In other cases, priapism may persist for days or even weeks and could lead to impotence. Some men find themselves enduring a painless enlargement of the penis that lasts for much greater lengths of time, perhaps years, and these men are usually impotent; they might occasionally suffer episodes of painful priapism for shorter periods of time on top of their more chronic condition.

The brain is the center of perception, learning, memory, and behavior—the seat of personhood. It is the central nervous system's command-and-control center. Different regions of the brain are headquarters for different functions, so the consequence of any failure of oxygen delivery depends on where in the brain the failure occurs and how extensive it is. The brain accounts for about 20 percent of the body's oxygen consumption. Its need for a constant adequate blood supply is absolute. The red blood cells of sickle cell patients carry less oxygen than normal red blood cells do, and this difference is compensated for in the brain by the delivery of larger volumes of blood to it. In some people, the pressure this elevated volume produces appears to be a cause of severe headaches. Strokes occur when brain cells do not receive adequate oxygen, and this can bring about death or major disabilities. When younger children suffer strokes, they are usually caused by the blockage of some of the brain's blood vessels. In older children and adults, strokes usually originate from the bleeding of blood vessels within the brain. Strokes can result in paralysis of one side of the body or in the loss of feeling on one side. Sometimes patients undergo convulsions or slip into coma, and some suffer visual impairment or lose their ability to speak. These symptoms might appear suddenly or gradually, and recovery might be fast or slow, partial or apparently complete. Strokes tend to recur often, but when chronic blood transfusions are given, perhaps every three to four weeks, the likelihood of recurrence is greatly reduced.

Gallstones

It has already been mentioned that a by-product of red cell destruction is bilirubin, a pigment that is excreted by the liver into the bile. Because so many red blood cells are destroyed in sickle cell disease, bilirubin is produced in very high amounts, and excess bilirubin leads to the formation of gallstones. These gallstones are small stones containing mostly bilirubin and also calcium, phosphates, cholesterol, and bile salts; they form in the gallbladder or bile passages. With sickle cell disease, gallstones form even in very young children, and the likelihood of producing gallstones increases with age. When gallstones are accompanied by symptoms, surgical removal of the gallbladder is usually the recommended treatment. This surgery has little consequence, however, because people do very well without their gallbladders. Gallstones may produce no symptoms at all or they may cause chronic problems, such as a bloating discomfort after eating, nausea, vomiting, and mild abdominal pain, or they may cause acute problems, such as fever, chills, and severe pain. The symptoms are due to inflammation or to obstruction of the ducts that bile travels through, and their severity depends on the size and number of the stones, where they have lodged, and the damage they have done. The problems get worse if infection sets in.

Psychological Aspects

Another important aspect of sickle cell disease is its psychological effects. Sickle cell disease is similar to other chronic diseases in the emotional impact it has on both the individual and the family. Sickle cell children must separate from their families during hospital stays, and some children fear that they are being abandoned. Severe pain, isolation, and disability take a psychological toll, and anxiety is common. For some, there is a haunting fear of death.

Sickle cell children are often smaller and thinner than their peers, they look different, and some may find themselves less intellectually competent. Many have lost time from school and suffer the academic consequences. As a result, sickle cell children and adolescents may have low self-esteem. They may become socially withdrawn. Some may suffer depression, and depression seems to be associated with episodes of pain. Adolescents and adults may become dependent on drugs, or even addicted to them. Sickle cell adults face thoughts of death and dying and a possible decrease of intellectual ability. Sickle cell disease patients need sound and robust emotional support (Chapter 5).

A Life Cycle

The complications of sickle cell disease discussed above were organized according to their nature and the parts of the body they affect. Below, they are reorganized in terms of a lifetime and what can be expected when. Again, not every sickle cell person will display every complication of the disease. Some complications, such as back and limb pain, are very common; others, such as acute splenic sequestration, are rare.

Infancy. Prior to birth, both normal and sickle cell disease fetuses make Hb F. After birth, Hb F production is replaced by Hb A production in healthy babies and by Hb S production in sickle cell babies. (Although Hb A is generally referred to as "adult" hemoglobin, it would be more accurate to refer to it as "after birth" hemoglobin.) During early infancy, depending on how long it takes for Hb S to become the dominant form, the baby with sickle cell disease is usually without symptoms. Infections usually start after two to three months, but many children remain symptom-free for a year or more. In the absence of prophylactic antibiotics, children die of infection between the ages of one and three years. As screening of the newborn becomes more prevalent, such early deaths will decrease.

Early childhood. Hand-foot syndrome is often the first problem to present itself. Infections, especially of the lungs and kidney, begin to occur at the same time, although their incidence can be modified by prophylactic antibiotics. Pneumococcal septicemia is one of the more common problems. Infections are often associated with painful episodes. Painful episodes can produce organ damage. By age two, the child usually has an enlarged spleen and there is a danger of splenic sequestration. Other problems common to early childhood include anemia and gallstones. Occasionally, young boys suffer episodes of priapism.

Mid to late childhood. Splenic sequestration and hand-foot syndrome usually are not problems for children after the age of five, and infections become less frequent by age ten. Strokes, which were not very common in the very first years of life, increase in frequency. Strokes can affect intellectual ability, eyesight, speech, and the ability to move or to sense the environment, and they can bring death. Priapism, too, increases in frequency in later childhood. Painful episodes (and accompanying organ damage) become more problematic. Physical growth is retarded. Since the nutritional demands of massive red blood cell production and constant tissue repair may not be met by most diets, this slow growth could be due to undernourishment.

Adolescence. On entering adolescence, sickle cell children find themselves smaller, lighter, and less sexually developed than their peers. The bodily hair patterns signaling maturity are late in coming for both sexes, and boys may have smaller testicles than their peers and correspondingly lower levels of the hormone testosterone. Girls may lag a year or more behind their peers in the onset of menstruation and breast development. Menstruation is more likely to be painful and less likely to be regular. Nevertheless, pregnancy is achievable for the adolescent girl with sickle cell disease.

A manifestation of sickle cell disease that becomes frequent in adolescence, especially in boys, is leg ulceration; in addition to being painful and a potential source of infection, these open sores tend to interfere with social activities and employment opportunities. Painful episodes become more common in adolescence, and hip-joint injury may become extensive enough to curtail ordinary activities and necessitate surgery or the use of crutches. Bed-wetting is common, and priapism often painfully disrupts sleep.

Adulthood. Painful episodes and leg ulcerations become less frequent for adults. Strokes, which were most common in early childhood, re-emerge as a threat in the third decade of life. In the kidney, injuries and scarring accumulated over the years lessen the organ's ability to function. Chronic kidney failure causes illness and death increasingly with age. Heart failure may strike the sickle cell adult, and in some cases the causes are not understood.

Pregnancy. Pregnancy used to present a major risk to women with sickle cell disease. Maternal mortality rates have declined steadily over the years, however, and today, the maternal death rate is very low. Prenatal care beginning early in pregnancy is strongly recommended.

Because she is not starting out in top-notch condition, the expectant mother with sickle cell disease may not thrive with the added physical demands of pregnancy. *Toxemia of pregnancy* (various physiological disturbances that cause symptoms ranging from high blood pressure to convulsions and coma), *thrombophlebitis* (inflammation of veins following formation of blood clots within them), kidney disease, heart failure, and spontaneous abortions—complications of pregnancy that occur in the normal population—occur with greater frequency in the sickle cell population. In addition, anemia, bone pain, and chest pain—symptoms that are common in sickle cell disease— become more common in pregnancy. The medically cared-for patient will usually receive folic acid and iron supplements to reduce anemia (provided it is not caused by infection or bleeding). Treatment for all the various expressions of sickle cell disease generally remain the same in pregnancy, including the administration of pain-killing drugs when it is called for.

The *placenta* (the newly formed organ that transmits oxygen and nourishment from the mother's blood to the fetus's and waste products from the fetus's blood to the mother's), with its numerous tiny blood vessels and sinusoids and its high oxygen needs, is particularly vulnerable to blood flow blockage. In late pregnancy, other organs commonly undergo blood vessel blockage, including the lungs, kidneys, and brain. Even in the face of such problems, sickle cell mothers can have successful pregnancies, and increasingly more are doing so. The maternal death rate has become almost negligible among those who receive proper prenatal care. A little bonus comes from the sickle cell woman's tendency to give birth prematurely: the low-birth-weight infants they tend to produce generally make for an easy delivery.

A Word About Sickle Cell Trait

People with sickle cell trait are very much like people with two Hb A genes. They live as long, and they are not hospitalized any more often. They do not have episodes of sickle cell disease unless they are subject to extreme oxygen deprivation. People with sickle cell trait do occasionally display symptoms, however. Some cannot produce concentrated urine and, as a result, need to urinate frequently. Some may find blood in their urine now and then; this is caused by sickling in the kidneys and is not associated with painful episodes. Sometimes sickling occurs in the spleen and, very rarely, in other organs. All in all, however, people with sickle cell trait lead normal lives. For responsible individuals with sickle cell trait, the only thing to worry about is family planning (Chapter 6).

5. How to Care for People with Sickle Cell Disease

The lives of sickle cell people have improved dramatically over the past two decades because our understanding of the disease has improved dramatically. Although understanding the disease has not yet brought a cure, it has enabled us to decrease its dangers and ease its pain. Timely medical care is an absolute essential for the well-being of sickle cell patients, but so is knowledgeable home care. Home care starts when the sickle cell child is an infant. The important first step is to find out as early as possible whether a child has, or is going to have, sickle cell disease. Today, this is easy. The disease can be diagnosed before birth (see Chapter 6) as well as after (see below), and the chance of conceiving a sickle cell child can usually be predicted even before conception (see Chapter 1).

Sickle cell screening programs for newborn infants exist in forty of the United States and in Puerto Rico and the Virgin Islands. In 1987, a conference held at the National Institutes of Health concluded that universal screening (the screening of all newborns) should be mandated by state laws so that treatment can be started in infancy. As of 1994, universal screening was provided in thirty-four states. Parents from sickle cell families can call their local board of health, their regional network for genetics services, or their state genetics services coordinators to find out where they can have their infant tested for sickle cell disease or how they can gain access to a sickle cell disease program (see Appendix).

Infant screening is done with blood samples collected at birth from the umbilical cord or from a heel prick. These blood samples are analyzed to see what kinds of hemoglobin the infant produces. If commercial laboratories do the testing, the procedures they should use are *hemoglobin electrophoresis, iso-electric focusing,* or *high performance liquid chromatography.* Two tests that should not be relied upon are the *metabisulfite test* and the *solubility test*; these are not sensitive enough. When abnormal hemoglobin is found, the physician may then want to have the DNA of the sample analyzed for a genetic diagnosis. Often, the testing procedure is repeated—starting with a new blood sample—to make sure that the results are accurate.

After a sickle cell diagnosis, arrangements for continuous medical care should be made with a physician or a sickle cell program. This should be done immediately after birth so that treatment can begin at the appropriate time, which will be very soon. Taking the child for regular medical check-ups and understanding the doctor's instructions are serious responsibilities. The focus of this chapter is not medical care, however, but home care, and that is the next step—to learn how to provide home care and support for the growing sickle cell child. Children with sickle cell disease have special needs that family, friends, and teachers can meet, once they know how.

One of the family's first responsibilities is to understand and comply with the physician's instructions. Care-givers will be expected to provide a *proper diet, adequate fluids, prescribed medications, appropriate day-to-day care,* and *a watchful eye.* Sickle cell children commonly suffer painful episodes, and sometimes the pain may be too severe to be relieved at home. When this happens, the family should understand the role of drugs in pain relief (see *Severe Pain,* p.74). In addition, children growing up with sickle cell disease need robust psychological support.

Proper diet. The nutritional demands of children during periods of accelerated growth are legendary. Some adolescents seem to stop eating only for sleep and dental care. Sickle cell children undergo growth spurts just as their healthy peers do, but their bodies make additional demands that divert nutrients away from growth. The food these children eat is used first to make new red blood cells (they need to replace the damaged cells that are continually being destroyed). Sickle cell children also have higher metabolic rates than their peers, which further increases their need for calories. Thus, they should be encouraged to eat a balanced, high calorie diet with sufficient protein. This way, their growth will not be limited by inadequate nutrition. The child's physician may also recommend dietary supplements of vitamins or minerals. Even with the best of nutrition, sickle cell children are likely to remain slim and, for a while at least, smaller than their healthy peers, so there's no point in constantly encouraging them to eat more.

Adequate fluids. There was a discussion in Chapter 3 on the factors that tend to cause red blood cells to sickle. One of these was a high Hb S concentration. The more concentrated Hb S is, the closer the Hb S molecules are to each other and the more likely they are to come into contact with each other. Once the Hb S molecules make contact, they polymerize. When fluids enter the red blood cell they dilute Hb S, lessening the likelihood of the molecules coming into contact with each other and polymerizing. That is one reason why sickle cell people need to drink generous amounts of fluid every day. Another is to keep the blood less viscous, which helps it to flow.

Since children with sickle cell disease are usually more thirsty than their healthy peers, it is easy to encourage them to drink a lot. Any clear fluids will do—water, milk, fruit juices, soft drinks, ices, popsicles, gelatin, and of course, chicken soup. There are certain times when sickle cell people should be encouraged to drink even more than they might care to. One such time is when they are experiencing pain. Pain suggests that blood vessels are clogging somewhere, and additional fluid might help the blood to flow again. Fever is another reason to encourage drinking. Fever could be due to blood vessel blockage or it could be due to infection, a real troublemaker (Chapter 4). In either case, fever causes the body to lose water through the skin. To make the blood more fluid and to help prevent Hb S polymerization, the lost water should be replaced by an increased intake of fluids.

Other situations that require increased fluid intake are any that cause water loss. These include diarrhea, hot weather, dry hot rooms, and strenuous activity such as sports and active play. For these conditions, and for pain and fever, there is a guide that can be used for fluid intake: Children weighing up to 35 pounds should consume a cup of fluid for every five pounds of their weight each day; larger children should consume a cup of fluid for every six pounds of their weight each day. On a very hot day, for example, a 15-pound child should be given about three cups of fluid (15 ÷ 5), and a 65-pound child should be encouraged to drink ten to eleven cups of fluid (65 ÷ 6).

Prescribed medications. Not very long ago, sickle cell children died at a very young age because they could not fight infections (Chapter 4). Today, sickle cell children are given antibiotics to fight infections for them. Penicillin is the antibiotic that is usually prescribed, generally when children are about two months of age. Erythromycin may be prescribed for those allergic to penicillin. Contrary to their usual use, antibiotics are given to sickle cell children to *prevent* infection, and they are given every day, twice a day, *no matter how healthy the child feels.* The usual dose is 125 milligrams[13] twice a day until the child is three years of age. Then the dose is usually increased to 250 milligrams twice a day, until the doctor says it is time to stop. (Older children and adults are not given prophylactic antibiotics.)

Penicillin comes in pills and in liquid form. The pills are more convenient because they last longer, do not spill, and do not need to be kept cold (the liquid does). The only problem with pills is that young children cannot swallow them. A good way to solve this problem is to crush the pill and mix it with a bit of food (chocolate ice cream, for example). The crushed pills could also be placed in drinks, but that would require careful watching to make sure that all the drink gets drunk. If liquid penicillin is used, it can be given from a spoon or from a dropper. As with the crushed penicillin pills, it is better not to place the liquid penicillin in a drink because drinks are often not finished. If a child has too much difficulty taking the penicillin, there is still recourse: the antibiotic can be given by injection in a doctor's office; this would be done every three weeks or so.

Penicillin, however, is not effective against all infections, nor does it give lifetime protection, so sickle cell children still need to receive the regular immunizations their peers receive—protection against diphtheria, whooping cough, tetanus, polio, measles, mumps, rubella, and any other the physician recommends.

Appropriate day-to-day care. Eating properly, drinking plenty of fluids, and following medical care plans are the basics of a sound day-to-day routine for sickle cell children, and for adults as well. So is avoiding alcohol, tobacco, and illegal drugs (as it is for anyone else). Temperature extremes should be avoided. Extreme heat causes *dehydration* (the loss of body fluids) and means that extra liquids must be consumed. Extreme cold can bring on painful episodes, although no one really understands why (Chapter 4). Care must be taken to make sure that sickle cell people stay warm when their surroundings are cold. Swimming in unheated water is not a good idea, but sports in general and other physical activities are fine. Sickle cell children do not usually have the strength or stamina to engage in athletic activities in a competitive way. By pacing themselves, however, and by taking time out when they feel tired (even if they are winning), they can still be physically active. Activities at high altitudes, such as hiking and skiing, can cause some people problems because the air at high altitudes contains less oxygen, and this could bring about sickling (Chapter 3).

Sickle cell children should follow the same day-to-day practices when they are away from home. Therefore teachers, coaches, scout leaders, daycare workers, baby-sitters, travel companions, and all other adults involved with them should be made part of a knowledgeable care-giving team. They should be told of the special needs of sickle cell children, how to deliver routine care, when to seek medical help (see *A watchful eye*, p.73), and the importance of psychological and social support (see *Psychological Support*, p.75).

Because of the connection between stress and painful episodes, sickle cell people should be protected from stress as much as possible. Parents should be tuned in to the kind of situations and environments that bring about painful episodes so that they can help their child avoid them. Pain itself is a source of stress, and managing a child's pain is a major responsibility. When painful episodes are mild, they are best treated in the home setting. First, sources of stress should be removed and efforts made to relax the child and ease its anxieties. Some children respond best to bedrest. Others are more comforted by quiet play or engaging activities, such as reading or being read to, listening to music, or watching television. (Extra fluids should be offered at the same time.) Second, efforts should be made to ease the pain by increasing blood flow. Warm baths often help. Or heat can be applied to the painful area. A heating pad can be used for this, or a towel that has been immersed in hot water and then wrung out; after the towel cools down, it can be replaced with a freshly warmed one. Another technique is to massage the area gently (it is helpful to first apply warm lotion or baby oil to the palms of the hands). Some older patients have learned to relieve their pain through training in special psychological techniques such as *thermal biofeedback* and *self-hypnosis*.

Medicine can also be used in the home to relieve sickle cell pain. The medicine could be acetaminophen (Tylenol, Tempra, or Panadol), aspirin, or a weak narcotic (such as codeine, oxycodone, or propoxyphene), whichever the physician recommends. Doses depend on the size of the child. It is important that mild pain be dealt with promptly. If it isn't, the pain can become more severe and more difficult to control, bringing with it more stress and more anxiety. Severe pain is generally not managed in the home setting (see *Severe Pain*, p.74).

A watchful eye. It has already been mentioned that caregivers should take note of the circumstances and environments that seem to bring about painful episodes so that children can be protected from them as much as possible. Care-givers should also watch for physical signs of trouble. They should learn to determine which problems can be dealt with at home, which should prompt a phone call to the doctor, and which require an immediate trip to the doctor's office or a hospital.

A major childhood danger is infection, and a clue for the presence of infection is fever. A thermometer for monitoring fever should be kept accessible everywhere a sickle cell child spends time. (Rectal thermometers are usually used for the very young, oral thermometers for everyone else. The new digital thermometers can be used orally or rectally or even under the armpit, and they do the job quickly.) Normal body temperature is 98.6° Fahrenheit (37° Celsius in the metric system). The doctor should be called when a sickle cell child has a fever of 101° F (38.3° C) or more. If the doctor cannot be reached, the child should be taken to a hospital emergency room. Other times to arrange immediate medical attention for sickle cell children are when they complain of severe headaches or dizziness, chest pain, or severe stomach pain; when they have trouble breathing or painful erections; and when they display a swollen abdomen, loss of color, seizures, weakness, paralysis, or an inability to wake up. These are the danger signs that require immediate

There are other problems that may not be
\ould nevertheless prompt a call to the physi-
\ repeated vomiting or diarrhea, jaundice,
nny or stuffed nose, unusual behavior, and
... ﹖ eat or drink or to take antibiotics.

Even closer attention must be paid to newborn babies and
infants since they are not able to communicate their distress. A
newborn baby or infant should be brought to a doctor quickly
if it is breathing rapidly or having a problem with breathing; if
it coughs frequently, is cranky, cries more than usual, or
screams when touched; if it is very weak or very tired or has little energy; if it does not want to eat, vomits, or has diarrhea; if
it has fewer wet diapers, pain or swelling in the abdomen,
swollen hands or feet, or pale blue or grey lips or skin.

When a child is brought to a hospital emergency room, the
emergency staff cannot be expected to know that the child has
sickle cell disease; they must be told, and the specific problem
must be explained. All care-givers should become familiar with
the list of symptoms that indicate it is time to get immediate
medical help or to call for advice.

Severe Pain

Severe pain that cannot be relieved at home is usually managed in the hospital with strong narcotics such as morphine.
Physicians, parents, and patients are sometimes concerned
about the use of strong narcotics because they worry about the
possibility of addiction. This concern is not supported by evidence, however. In studies of tens of thousands of hospitalized
adults, including burn victims, cancer patients, and patients re-
covering from surgery, the relief of pain by narcotics did not
cause addiction. While addiction does develop in people who
take narcotics for its psychological effects, people who take
them for the relief of pain rarely become "hooked" unless they
have abused drugs in the past or have psychological problems

to begin with. Moreover, those seeking pain relief do not re-quire the ever-increasing doses that addicts require. They may need gradually increasing doses at first, but the effective, pain-relieving dose soon becomes stable. In hospital studies, when patients in pain were put in control of their own narcotics doses (by pushing a button causing morphine to be injected into a vein), they did not develop drug dependence, but low-ered their doses as their pain diminished.

There will always be some people who prefer to "tough it out," but withholding narcotics from a person seeking relief from severe pain may be unjustified and even cruel. According to guidelines on acute pain management put out by the Agency for Health Care Policy and Research, children are likely to talk less about pain than adults, so the burden of vigilance for pain rests with the health care provider. The guidelines, which were not developed for disease pain but for children undergoing painful medical procedures such as surgery, affirm "the rights of all children in any institution to receive the best level of pain relief that can be provided safely." They note that there are no studies of the risks of addiction in children, but "no known as-pect of childhood development or physiology increases the risk of physiologic or psychologic chemical dependence."[14]

For patients living in the less savory neighborhoods of big cities like New York, there is another concern. Children see drug addicts almost daily and witness what terrible people they are. They fear that they, too, may become terrible people if they take drugs. Parents should try to allay such fears, explaining the difference between drugs for therapy and drugs for recre-ation.

Psychological Support

Afflicted children experience periods of relatively good health interspersed with periods of illness. As medical prob-lems present themselves, they can be handled by physicians and other trained professionals. There is another dimension to sickle cell disease, however, that must be handled by the family itself, and that is the behavioral, social, and psychological effects of the illness on everyone involved.

The first people to face psychological difficulties in the sickle cell family are the parents of the afflicted child. When parents learn that they have a sickle cell child, they sometimes respond in ways that hinder their ability to deal with the situation. For example, they may feel disbelief, anxiety, anger, hostility, or depression. They may also feel guilty because they know the child inherited the disease from them. When such feelings persist, they can interfere with the ability of parents to seek information and provide the proper care for their child. Sickle cell disease, however, is not the fault of the child, of the parents, or of the parents' parents; it is an accident of nature that survived and persists because, as we have seen, the sickle cell gene did something good for people that lived in another place at another time (Chapter 2). Parents who need help coping with their child's condition should ask about programs in their community where they can get counseling. Some parents feel strengthened by participation in a *support group*, where they can meet with other parents of sickle cell children. Both sickle cell programs and local support groups can help parents deal with their feelings, and they can also provide them with the information they need to go about sickle cell parenting in a sensible and knowledgeable way (see *Support Groups*, p.79).

Healthy brothers and sisters of a sickle cell child may also have psychological problems. They might not receive the share of attention they would normally expect or the amount they think they need. They may resent all the attention shown the afflicted child. Moreover, since the illness may produce a drain on the family's energy and money, these children may lose out on trips or toys or family play or fancy shoes or other things they might otherwise enjoy. Therefore, the parents of sickle cell children need to engage in a difficult balancing act, paying attention to each child while providing special protection—but not too much of it—to the sickle cell child.

Parents minister to sickle cell children with constant vigilance—observing their behavior, watching for fever, pain, or fatigue, dispensing medications, and monitoring nutrition and fluid intake. If parents are overprotective, however, it can be psychologically hurtful. Overprotection reinforces helpless and dependent behavior in the growing child, and it reduces the child's *self-esteem* (feeling good about oneself). Knowing parents, therefore, treat the child "normally." They try to deal with the sickle cell child's behavior as they would the behavior of any other child. Although their health care needs are special, sickle cell children, like healthy children, should be held to behavioral standards, given responsibility, and judiciously disciplined. They should be encouraged to develop interests, friends, and hobbies. They should be enrolled in school and expected to perform there to the best of their ability. When school days are missed, efforts should be made to help the sickle cell child keep up. The teacher can be asked to send home material so that a parent or a friend can provide instruction at home. Such upbringing helps the child to develop into a socially responsible individual, one that gets along well with others and interacts comfortably in the school setting. Social acceptance and pride of performance help all people feel good about themselves, and they reduce emotional stress; this is especially important for sickle cell children, because for them, emotional stress and pain feed on each other.

Children who adjust best to sickle cell disease are those who have ample self-esteem, understand their disease, feel in control of their own lives, and come from strongly bonded families. Family efforts, therefore, should be made to help sickle cell children feel useful, productive, worthwhile, knowledgeable about their disease, and increasingly in control of their lives. One way to help children feel more in control would be to entrust them with some part of the management of their disease; medications would be one example. In addition, they could learn why the medication is given and study how it works. They might find satisfaction in obtaining more detailed information about sickle cell disease. They could begin to read more extensively, and, if they like, become experts in sickle cell biology. But even within a caring and dependable family unit, the sickle cell child may harbor conflicting feelings. Although afflicted children love and need their families, they may also hate their parents for giving them sickle cell disease, and they may resent their normal brothers and sisters for the carefree lives they lead. Parents should not be shocked by such feelings; patient understanding would be more appropriate.

Adolescence, the time for accelerated independence and adult aspirations, is a problem for sickle cell children who have difficulty envisioning a life of independence and accomplishment. The body may reshape itself for adult functions (albeit later than for normal peers), but the sickle cell adolescent may feel neither attractive nor sexually adequate. Moreover, this new body is still a source of unpredictable pain. (Some communities have adolescent sickle cell support groups that help adolescents work these feelings out.) Sickle cell adolescents may fear competition with their healthy peers. They may fear difficulty in getting jobs because of poor academic records that follow from school absences. And the jobs they would be able to hold would necessarily be limited. Since those jobs should not be too physically demanding, the development of more sedentary interests and skills—perhaps through college attendance or career training—could prepare sickle cell adolescents for employment suited to them. Sickle cell adolescents worry that if they cannot get a good job, they will not be able to take care of themselves. And how can they date? Or marry? The problems facing the adolescent range from formidable to terrifying. Nevertheless, many sickle cell people have survived adolescence with sufficient personal resources and emotional strength to successfully separate themselves from their families, to form healthy peer relationships, to say "I'm OK," and even to say "I do."

Pregnancy could present a major risk to the sickle cell female and to her fetus as well. It is therefore important for adolescents and women with sickle cell disease to avoid unwanted pregnancies. This requires total commitment. Fertile girls and women who do not want to become pregnant have only two choices: to *never* engage in sexual intercourse, or to *always* practice contraception. Nothing else works. Chapter 6 discusses the various birth-control options available. When a sickle cell woman thinks she may be pregnant, she should visit her doctor or clinic right away. The doctor will request regular and frequent visits, perhaps weekly ones, and will provide instructions on proper diet, activities, and nutritional supplements. In addition, the doctor can test the father's blood to find out whether he, too, produces abnormal hemoglobin. If he does, *prenatal* (prior to birth) *testing* of the fetus can determine whether it is destined to have sickle cell disease. If it is, the expectant parents might want to discuss their options with their physician or a genetics counselor (see Chapter 6).

Support Groups

In peer support groups, people who have sickle cell disease may develop more positive attitudes and more effective coping strategies. Peer support groups provide opportunities for affected families and friends to talk with others experiencing the same medical problems, to share stories of success and failure, to learn about available resources, and, most importantly, to meet others who can truthfully say, "I understand; I know how you feel," based on their own experiences. In parent support groups, information about the disease is provided, and parents may develop ways to deal with some of their problems together. They may, for example, provide transportation services, or they may engage in fundraising to provide scholarships or training and vocational services. Some parent groups, recognizing that people with sickle cell disease may not do well in the traditional workplace, guide their youngsters toward entrepreneurial skills. Support groups usually form as part of a local chapter of the Sickle Cell Disease Association of America. People who want to form support groups in their own communities should contact the Association for help (see Appendix).

6. Planning a Family

No activity is more fundamental to human societies than creating families. Rituals, rules, and beliefs controlling reproductive behavior are found in every social group. These range from one extreme to the other. While some societies penalize a woman for having more than one child, other societies promote perpetual pregnancy. While some societies kill newborn babies just for being the wrong sex (that means female), other societies spend thousands of dollars a day to prolong the life of any baby, even one that has no brain. In the multicultural United States, there are many reproductive options available. This enables people of different beliefs to choose what is best for them. The purpose of this chapter is to provide information on family-planning choices available for couples at risk of transmitting sickle cell disease to their children.

The ultimate goal of sickle cell research is a cure for the disease. Until one is devised, the powerful tools of molecular biology are being used in the planning of families free of sickle cell disease. Some countries with high hemoglobin disease rates have been doing this for years; they have greatly improved the lives of at-risk families and at the same time have reduced national health care costs. In the 1970s, some Mediterranean countries used the mass media (television, newspapers, etc.) to launch voluntary public health programs designed to reduce the number of children born with hemoglobin disorders. As a consequence of these programs, the frequency of children born with a severe form of beta thalassemia (a disease associated with severe anemia, marked wasting, and early death) in Italy, Greece, and Cyprus went down from 1 per 250 births to 1 per 1,000 births. Ninety percent of severe thalassemia cases were prevented. The same techniques are available in this country, but the prevention of sickle cell births has not become part of an aggressive national public health program.

In the United States, as in the above Mediterranean countries, women can voluntarily eliminate the risk of having sickle cell children and still raise families. Currently, about 1000 sickle cell babies are born in the United States each year. Using modern family planning techniques, the odds of having a sickle cell child that were calculated in Chapter 1 can be overcome, with one exception. Except when both partners are afflicted (this was case 1 in Chapter 1), at-risk couples can plan their families so that none of their children will be born with sickle cell disease. Prospective parents who do not know whether they are at risk for having sickle cell children (see Chapter 1) can request genetic testing to learn if they carry Hb S genes. Local health departments generally know where genetic testing can be done. State genetic services coordinators also have this information. There are genetic services coordinators in every state as well as in the District of Columbia, Puerto Rico, and the Virgin Islands; their phone numbers are listed in the Appendix.

Couples who want to speak to a knowledgeable person about their risk and what they can do about it should seek the services of a *genetic counselor*. Genetic counselors make sure that couples fully understand the possible outcomes of a pregnancy. They discuss what resources are required to raise an afflicted child and what its life would probably be like. They explain available options should a sickle cell pregnancy occur. Professional genetic counselors, however, do not direct decisions; they only provide the information needed to make those decisions. What kind of family to have is left to the couple to decide. Couples who want to find a genetic counselor should contact their local sickle cell screening programs or their local genetic services coordinator (see Appendix). With or without a genetics counselor, couples who know they can transmit sickle cell disease need to decide whether they want to avoid having sickle cell children. If couples decide that they *do* want to avoid having sickle cell children, they have three options: (1) they can avoid pregnancy completely, (2) they can aim for pregnancy, have prenatal testing done on the fetus, and only complete those pregnancies that promise a healthy outcome, or (3) they can request *pre-implantation diagnosis* procedures.

Option 1 is technically the easiest and option 3 is technically the most advanced, but it is option 2—completing only non-sickle cell pregnancies—that is the most problematic in the United States today. And the problems are emotional, not technical. Some people profoundly believe that it is wrong to terminate a pregnancy; other people profoundly believe that it is wrong to bring into the world a child who is destined for suffering and pain. How couples deal with option 2 depends on their personal and religious beliefs. These generally vary with ethnic origin. Dr. D. J. Weatherall, Professor of Clinical Medicine at the University of Oxford (England), relates the following:[15]

> It is interesting to consider current attitudes to prenatal diagnosis for the hemoglobin disorders in different countries. Surprisingly, these programs have been widely accepted in predominantly Catholic countries such as Sardinia and Italy; I suspect this reflects the emergence of a more secular society rather than any change of attitude by the Church. While ethnic and religious objections to prevention of genetic disease by direct intervention seem to be becoming less common in many western countries, the situation is not nearly so clear in other parts of the world, particularly those with large Islamic populations. Indeed, from personal discussions it appears that there may be serious difficulties in setting up major prenatal diagnosis programs, at whatever age of gestation, in many Islamic countries. On the other hand, from experiences in Thailand, it seems that the largely Buddhist population will have less difficulty in accepting selective abortion, particularly if it is carried out early in pregnancy and if a good case for the mother's well-being can be made.

Unlike so many other countries, the United States, founded by immigrants, is a nation of mixed origins. We have all of the

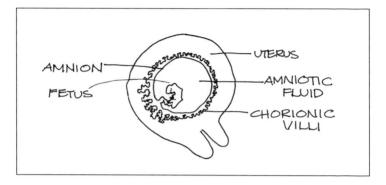

FIG. 6.1 The embryo and its membranes

ethnic groups mentioned above, and many more. The three options, which are described below, include something for everyone.

Avoiding Pregnancy

Two choices are available to couples who decide to have no biological children: contraception and sterilization. Contraception can be accomplished with pills or various devices. The advantage of contraception is that its action is not permanent; the disadvantage is that it is not perfect. Sometimes contraceptives fail, and sometimes people fail to use their contraceptives. A physician or family-planning clinic can advise individuals and couples about the various birth control techniques and the effectiveness of each. The last section of this chapter (Contraception for the Woman with Sickle Cell Disease) contains information that is relevant to women in general.

Unlike contraception, sterilization is usually nonreversible. Sterilization of either partner will permanently prevent conception by that partner. It is only necessary for one partner to undergo sterilization so long as no other sexual partnerships are formed by the fertile person. Males who want to be sterile commonly undergo *vasectomy* (cutting of the tubes that move sperm from the testes toward the penis). Vasectomy does not require hospitalization and is done with local anaesthesia. It does not affect a man's sexual activity. Vasectomy has a negligible rate of failure. Females seeking sterilization commonly undergo cutting of the *fallopian tubes*. These tubes carry eggs to the uterus (womb), and it is in them that the eggs are fertilized. This surgery is commonly done through a tiny cut in the abdomen (at the navel) and is barely visible when it heals. The procedure does not require hospitalization and can be done with local or general anaesthesia. It normally does not affect a woman's sexual activity. It has a failure rate of 1 in 500.

Completing Pregnancies with a Healthy Outcome

Couples who decide they want to raise a family but do not want to bring a sickle cell child into the world can request prenatal screening services from a family planning clinic or a private physician. Their personal family-planning program will involve prenatal diagnosis of sickle cell disease and, if it is their choice, early termination of a sickle cell pregnancy. Normal pregnancies would be carried to term. A woman who does not intend to terminate a pregnancy under any circumstances can still request prenatal diagnosis. A negative finding could eliminate worry, and a positive finding would enable her to better prepare for her sickle cell child.

Prenatal DNA Testing. Before DNA can be tested, a fetal tissue sample must be obtained. This is done by *chorionic villus sampling* or *amniocentesis*. As shown in figure 6.1, the embryo is surrounded by *amniotic fluid* and enclosed within two membranes. The inner membrane is the *amnion* and the outer membrane is the *chorion*. *Chorionic villi* are fingerlike projections that grow out of the chorion. These villi disappear later in embryonic development, except for the ones that penetrate the wall of the uterus and give rise to the placenta.

Fetal tissue is usually sampled from chorionic villi between about the ninth and fourteenth week of pregnancy. This is done by inserting either a needle through the abdomen or a thin tube through the vagina and cervix. The procedure is guided by *ultrasound*. (When ultrasound waves are directed at the fetus, it bounces the waves back, and these are used to produce a picture of the fetus on a television screen.) The advantage of chorionic villus sampling is that it can be done early in pregnancy and the results are usually accurate. The disadvantages include a slightly increased risk of fetal loss, a very slight increase in risk to the fetus of hand and foot birth defects, and a risk to the mother of some vaginal bleeding. As accurate as the procedure is, a wrong non-sickle cell diagnosis is still possible, especially by less experienced workers. The diagnosis can be checked again in the following trimester, however, by amniocentesis.

Amniocentesis (sampling of the amniotic fluid) is usually done between the fifteenth and twentieth weeks of pregnancy. A syringe, guided by ultrasound, is inserted through the abdomen into the amniotic sac and a sample of about four to six teaspoonfuls of fluid is removed for testing. There is a slight increase in fetal deaths associated with amniocentesis, and a low risk to the mother for inflammation of the amnion, vaginal bleeding, and amniotic fluid leakage.

Testing fetal DNA involves one of the most dazzling molecular techniques developed in recent years, the *polymerase chain reaction* (PCR). PCR makes it possible to take a tiny sample of DNA and make many, many copies of a selected portion of it so that there is ample DNA to test or work with. PCR uses nucleotides (the As, Ts, Gs, and Cs of Chapter 1), an enzyme (*polymerase*) that zips the nucleotides together to form new DNA, and a primer that shows the enzyme which DNA to make copies of. The portion copied for sickle cell diagnosis is a section of the beta globin gene containing the tell-tale code for the sixth amino acid (see Chapter 1 for a discussion of this).

PCR works in cycles, and the number of DNA copies is doubled with each cycle. Since we are starting with one cell, there are two copies of all the DNA to begin with. After one PCR cycle there would be four copies of the targeted DNA, and after two cycles there would be eight copies. After nine cycles, there would be 1,024 copies (try it). After nineteen cycles, there would be over a million copies. In actual practice, however, the number of copies produced is lower than the predicted number because the system is not perfect. Nevertheless, PCR can be used to produce enough DNA for an accurate diagnosis of sickle cell disease. There are several methods for making the diagnosis. The most commonly used methods employ DNA "probes." The probes are labeled (with fluorescent dyes, for example) so that they can be seen. In these techniques, sickle cell DNA is identified if it matches up with sickle cell DNA probes (As with Ts, Gs with Cs, etc., as described in Chapter 1), and nonsickle DNA is identified when it matches up with nonsickle DNA probes.

Termination of pregnancy. The earlier a pregnancy is terminated, the simpler the procedure is. This is because the fetus is very small—about one-half ounce at the twelfth week. It is also a safe procedure—safer than childbirth—and does not affect a woman's ability to become pregnant again. If the pregnancy is terminated after fifteen or sixteen weeks, the procedure is more complex and may take a whole day, or even two. It, too, is a relatively safe procedure and does not affect a woman's fertility.

A new procedure for terminating pregnancy without surgery involves Mifepristone (RU-486), a synthetic hormone developed in France. Mifepristone acts by blocking the action of *progesterone*, a hormone that maintains pregnancy. Without progesterone, a fetus cannot stay attached to the uterus. Mifepristone, taken as a pill, is followed two days later by an

injection of *prostaglandin*, a drug that makes the uterus con-
tract. Mifepristone (plus prostaglandin) can be used through
the seventh week of pregnancy. It has a success rate of 96 percent. U.S. clinical trials involving 2,000 women began in 1994,
and the drug is expected to become available in 1996.

Pre-implantation diagnosis

Pre-implantation diagnosis is an appropriate choice for couples who want to have healthy children but, because of personal or religious beliefs, are unwilling to terminate a pregnancy. Pre-implantation diagnosis, however, is an advanced
technique that is not yet widely available. Pre-implantation diagnosis is done before pregnancy begins. Eggs are removed
from the ovary and uterus, transferred to a laboratory dish, and
fertilized (if they are not already fertilized). Under all the right
conditions, the fertilized eggs will begin to divide. After an egg
divides into several cells, perhaps eight, one of the cells is removed for DNA analysis.[16] If the analysis shows that the embryo has not inherited sickle cell disease, the physician im-
plants it in the mother's uterus. Successful pregnancy is
achieved on about one out of three tries.

Contraception for the woman with sickle cell disease

Pregnancy presents a great physical challenge to the sickle
cell patient. Women and girls who have sickle cell disease and
who are concerned about their own well-being should take all
possible steps to avoid unwanted pregnancy, regardless of its
potential outcome. Infant and child care is a demanding responsibility, and even greater demands are placed on the sickle
cell mother if she gives birth to a sickle cell child. Sickle cell
women, therefore, need to seriously evaluate whether they want

to raise a family, and they need to make a conscious decision. If they do not, chance will make that decision for them, and chance seems to favor pregnancy.

The safest thing for women and girls who do not want to become pregnant to do is to postpone sexual intercourse. If they do become sexually active, sickle cell women should thoroughly educate themselves in contraceptive techniques and choose what is best for them. Then, they should practice that technique unfailingly. Advice on contraception can be obtained from private physicians, local or state health departments (most of which have family planning clinics), and family-planning organizations such as Planned Parenthood (see Appendix).

Currently, all the traditional methods used by women in general are considered safe for women with sickle cell disease. Except for condoms, they all require a physician's prescription or can be obtained at Planned Parenthood and other family planning clinics. *IUDs* (*intrauterine devices*) are physical materials that prevent conception when they are placed inside the uterus. These may pose a risk of bleeding and infection. *Oral contraceptives* ("*the pill*") are hormone mixtures that prevent pregnancy by preventing *ovulation*—the monthly release of an egg. Oral contraception is the most reliable contraceptive method currently available. Some oral contraceptives can be used as *"morning-after pills"* (actually, there's about 72 hours leeway). *Diaphragms* are physical barriers to conception that fit over the cervix. Diaphragms are most effective when they are used together with a sperm-killing preparation. *Condoms* are physical barriers to conception traditionally worn by the male, although a female condom is also available. Condoms are best made of latex, and they prevent conception by keeping the sperm packaged. They are more effective when they are used together with a sperm-killing foam. Although condoms are not the most reliable contraceptive around, they are easily obtained (in pharmacies, for example) and are the only known device that can protect against sexually transmitted diseases, including *AIDS* (*acquired immune deficiency syndrome*), *trichomoniasis,* and *gonorrhea.* Even sterile women and those protected from pregnancy by birth control pills should insist on condom use when there is the slightest possibility of contracting AIDS or other sexually transmitted diseases. (By the age of 21, one in five people in the United States requires treatment for a sexually transmitted disease.) Mifepristone, discussed above as a pregnancy-terminating agent, can also be used as a contraceptive. Technically, it does not prevent conception, but prevents embryos from attaching to the uterus. *Injectable contraceptives* are safe, effective, and widely used in some countries. The hormone *medroxyprogesterone,* which is injected every three months, has been reported to reduce the severity of sickle cell symptoms. This makes it a particularly attractive contraceptive method for sickle cell women.

Thus, there are many reproductive opportunites available for people in sickle cell families. Genetic testing is available for those who do not know their risk; a variety of effective contraceptive techniques are available for those who wish to avoid or postpone pregnancy; prenatal diagnosis, coupled with optional pregnancy termination, enables at risk couples to raise families without sickle cell disease; in vitro fertilization with pre-implantation diagnosis, where available, offers a high-tech route to non-sickle cell families that does not entail pregnancy termination; and genetic counseling provides at-risk couples with all the information they need to make their own family-planning decisions.

7. Searching for a Cure

Currently, people with sickle cell disease receive treatment for their symptoms, not a cure for their disease. Physicians and other care-givers prevent and manage infections, see that the nutritional demands of constant red cell replacement are met, and ease symptoms and pain as they arise. Such care is effective and improves the quality and length of life for sickle cell sufferers. The ultimate goal, however, is to prevent the symptoms from occurring in the first place. Research on a cure for sickle cell disease, or something close to a cure, is progressing along several different avenues. These include the following: (1) the development of anti-sickling agents, (2) turning on the genes that increase the production of Hb F, (3) bone marrow transplantation, and (4) gene therapy.

Anti-sickling agents. Different strategies are possible in the design of anti-sickling agents. One way to prevent sickling would be to prevent Hb S molecules from polymerizing on contact (Chapter 3). Drugs that accomplish this would need to concentrate in the red blood cell and interact with hemoglobin. Since there are so many hemoglobin molecules, large amounts of the drug would need to be taken. It would be important, therefore, for such drugs to be nontoxic. Although several potential anti-sickling agents have been screened over the years, they have not met the requirements of a good drug. Either they did not work as predicted or they were more harmful than helpful. One drug that did look somewhat promising is *vanillin*, a chemical found in the vanilla orchid as well as in other plants, and which can also be made in the laboratory. Vanillin concentrates in the red blood cell, interacts with hemoglobin, and inhibits polymer formation. It is now being studied in clinical trials.[17]

Another way to prevent sickling would be to dilute Hb S. As mentioned in Chapter 3, Hb S is less likely to polymerize when it is less concentrated. One way to dilute Hb S would be to change the nature of the red cell membrane so that the cell would hold more water. One such cell-swelling drug is *hydroxyurea*. Red cells made during hydroxyurea treatment appear to contain an increased amount of fluid. Also, the red blood cell population changes in a favorable way: the cells most likely to cause blood vessel clogging (the sticky ones and the irreversibly sickled ones) seem to disappear. Hydroxyurea is now being tested in clinical trials, but it is actually being tested because of a different effect (see section on Hb F, p. 93).

Other drugs interact with the red cell membrane and keep the cell more fluid and more flexible. Examples are *cetiedil* and *clotrimazole*. These drugs, however, have not undergone development by pharmaceutical companies.

Turning on the genes that increase the production of Hb F. Turning on the genes that increase the production of fetal hemoglobin is the idea that currently holds the most promise for sufferers of sickle cell disease. While it would not actually provide a cure, high levels of Hb F could inhibit sickling and its painful consequences. This technique should be approached with caution, however, because it is not specific for Hb F genes. Other genes might also be turned on, including genes that cause cancer.

The first suggestion that Hb F might have a protective effect in sickle cell disease came in 1948, when Dr. Janet Watson hypothesized that the reason sickle cell newborns did not have symptoms was that there were high Hb F levels in their red blood cells.[18] Subsequently it was discovered that sickle cell people who make larger amounts of Hb F often have a milder form of the disease. These include people with the Arab-Indian and Senegal haplotypes and people with mutations that cause them to continue to make Hb F as adults. (How Hb F exerts its protective effect is discussed in Chapter 3.) Such reports led scientists to wonder if increasing the amount of Hb F in sickle cell patients would make their disease less severe. To test this, they had to first figure out how to increase the amount of Hb F that sickle cell people make.

Reports from DNA research laboratories led scientists to suspect that the chemical *5-azacytidine* might work. Remember the letters of genetic alphabet—A, T, G, and C (Chapter 1)? The "C" stood for "cytosine." 5-Azacytidine looks very much like cytosine, so much so that DNA incorporates it in place of cytosine. When that happens, some genes that had been turned off, get turned on. When 5-azacytidine was tested in experimental animals (baboons), they made much more Hb F.

In the 1980s, 5-azacytidine was tried in some sickle cell disease patients. Soon these patients were making more Hb F. Over the clinical trial period (one to three years), the patients suffered less anemia and fewer painful episodes. In spite of this, the clinical trial was stopped because of evidence that the drug might cause cancer (it did so in rodents).

Another drug that has been tried is *hydroxyurea*. Hydroxyurea increases Hb F by suppressing bone marrow activity. When active marrow cells are suppressed, more of the less active marrow cells—the ones that make Hb F-producing cells—go into red cell production. Clinical trials with hydroxyurea have been progressing for several years and are still underway. The drug appears to work, but not uniformly and not in all patients. Those who do respond may experience fewer and milder painful episodes and enjoy improved general health. There is no way to tell in advance, however, who will respond and who will not. Hydroxyurea is also being tested clinically in combination with erythropoietin. As mentioned in Chapter 4, erythropoietin is a hormone that stimulates red blood cell production. When given in high doses, erythropoietin even stimulates the inactive stem cells (the ones that never shut off their Hb F genes) to produce red blood cells. When erythropoietin was given to baboons in high doses, the animals increased the amount of Hb F they made. When hydroxyurea and erythropoietin were given together, the effect was greater than the effect produced by either agent alone.

Another drug being investigated is *butyric acid*, a chemical found in milkfat and butter. In 1984, scientists reported that butyrate (together with 5-azacytidine, discussed above) turned on embryonic hemoglobin genes in adult chicken cells. Then it was reported that butyrate delayed the switching off of Hb F genes in fetal sheep; it also switched on the Hb F genes in adult baboons as well as in stem cells taken from sickle cell patients and grown in laboratory dishes. It was reported in 1985 that babies born to diabetic mothers had high Hb F levels. These infants also had high levels of butyric acid in their blood but were otherwise normal. It seemed likely that the high Hb F levels were caused by the butyric acid. In 1993, six children—three with sickle cell disease and three with thalassemia—were given daily injections of butyrate for three weeks. Investigators reported that an increase in Hb F followed and the children did not seem to be harmed by the treatment. Scientists are cautious, however, because the effects of long-term treatment are not known; baboons given long-term butyrate suffered from nerve damage, with symptoms that included drowsiness and loss of muscle coordination. Separate studies of two different forms of butyrates are now underway.

Bone marrow transplantation. For bone marrow transplantation, marrow cells donated by a person with normal hemoglobin are transplanted into a person with abnormal hemoglobin. Before receiving the marrow transplant, patients must take drugs that prevent immune reactions to the donor's cells. Since these drugs suppress immune responses to other foreign cells as well, treated patients are vulnerable to infection. The donor's cells, too, can have an immune reaction to the recipient. Because of these potential problems, transplantation can be performed only if a donor who is genetically very similar to the sickle cell patient, such as a close relative, is available. (Genetic similarity can be determined by testing.)

The advantage of this procedure is that it could bring about a true, long-term cure. The disadvantages are that it does not always work, and there can be serious immunologic complications. At this time, there is a 4 percent mortality rate. Because bone marrow transplantation is so dangerous, it is not often performed. In the future, however, it may become possible to look at a patient's genes and predict how severe his or her disease is likely to be. Then, the risks of the treatment could be weighed against the risks of the disease in deciding whether to try bone marrow transplantation. There would be little point in subjecting a person who is likely to have mild disease to such a dangerous treatment. On the other hand, bone marrow transplantation might be a good choice for a sickle cell child who is likely to suffer severe pain, serious disability, and early death.

Worldwide, bone marrow transplantation has been tried in forty-eight patients. Forty-seven of the donors were siblings (brothers or sisters) of the patients, and one was a parent. There were several complications, but the procedure was successful in forty-two of the patients. In the United States, bone marrow transplantation has been tried on five patients; marrow was donated by siblings. All five are alive and well at times ranging from eight months to over nine years since their treatment.

An immunologically less dangerous procedure that could be developed in the future is transplantation into a sickle cell individual while it is still a fetus. The advantage of this is that the fetal immune system does not develop until the second trimester. Thus, a first-trimester fetus would not recognize the donor's cells as foreign and would not react to them; no immuno-suppressive drugs would be needed. Ideally, the donor's cells also would not react to the recipient. One way to ensure this is to obtain donor stem cells from another (aborted) fetus;

another way is to use marrow from the mother after it has been treated to destroy its immune cells. Prenatal stem cell transplantation was reported in 1991.[19] Stem cells from an aborted 9-week-old fetus were injected into a 12-week-old fetus that had severe beta thalassemia. Although neither the mother nor the infant was harmed by the procedure, the thalassemia was not cured; it was determined after birth that the donor cells produced only a small fraction of the total blood cells. How to get the transplanted stem cells to grow in preference to the recipient's stem cells is not yet worked out. More research is needed before prenatal transplantation becomes a useful procedure.

Gene therapy. Gene therapy—transplanting "good" genes into people—is the ultimate cure for genetic diseases. Successful gene therapy would correct for the original genetic injury, and it would do so for a lifetime.[20] Gene therapy for sickle cell patients is a challenging, if not a daunting, process. First, copies of normal hemoglobin genes must be made. Then they must be inserted into the right kind of stem cells—and lots of them. Then these stem cells must be put back into the marrow. There, they must implant and produce red cells that make enough Hb A to prevent polymerization of the Hb S. Better still, the gene therapy would inactivate the Hb S gene.

Some of these procedures have been worked out. Hb A gene copies can be made by PCR (Chapter 6), they can be inserted into the stem cell by packaging them inside a virus that infects the cell, and the gene-treated marrow cells do implant themselves when they are put back into the host. A major problem remaining is that the re-implanted marrow cells do not produce adequate amounts of Hb A. Getting them to produce more is an active area of research. The treatment also has worrisome potential hazards: when the new gene inserts itself into the chromosome, there is as yet no way to be certain that it would not activate a cancer gene or inactivate an essential or cancer-suppressing gene. Because of these unknowns, it will be some time before gene therapy is used to treat sickle cell disease.

These, then, are the areas of research being pursued by scientists seeking a cure for sickle cell disease. It is difficult to know which will be the most fruitful, but there is no doubt that a cure, or something close to it, will be found.

In January 1995, a clinical trial of hydroxyurea (discussed earlier in this chapter) was terminated with dramatic results. The drug, which was given as a pill to adults with severe sickle cell disease, reduced by half the number of painful episodes, hospitalizations, situations requiring blood transfusions, and occurrences of acute chest syndrome. The National Institutes of Health, which supported the research, issued a clinical alert telling physicians that they should now consider using the drug—but not for children or for women planning to have children. The drug will be tested on children in a two-year clinical trial to begin soon. The long-term effects of hydroxyurea are still not known.

Appendix

Many resources are available for people seeking information on or treatment for sickle cell disease or strategies to prevent it in their children. Local phone directories usually list state or local boards of health, and these are good sources of information and assistance. The following organizations can also be helpful.

The Sickle Cell Disease Association of America (formerly the National Association For Sickle Cell Disease) is a voluntary non-profit organization. SCDAA supports research, education, screening, counselor training, and support and service programs. It publishes a quarterly newsletter (which you can receive free of charge) and other informational material. The national office is at 3345 Wilshire Boulevard, Suite 1106, Los Angeles, California 90010-1880. The toll-free number is 1-800-421-8453.

The **Federal Government** funds sickle cell disease programs through (1) the National Heart, Lung, and Blood Institute of the National Institutes of Health, and (2) the Bureau of Maternal and Child Health of the Health Resources and Services Administration.

1) The Sickle Cell Disease Branch of the National Heart, Lung, and Blood Institute funds ten **Comprehensive Sickle Cell Centers**. These provide education, testing, and counselling. Clinical and laboratory research are also conducted in these centers. NIH also funds additional sickle cell disease research in other laboratories throughout the United States. The NIH Comprehensive Sickle Cell Centers that have been established for 1993-1998, and their directors, are as follows:

Alabama
Steven R. Goodman, Ph.D.
College of Medicine
University of South Alabama
2451 Fillinghim Street
Mobile, AL 36617
(205) 460-7334

California
William C. Mentzer, M.D.
University of California
San Francisco General Hospital
1001 Potrero Avenue, Room 6J-5
San Francisco, CA 94110
(415) 206-5169

Cage S. Johnson, M.D.
Department of Medicine, RMR 304
University of Southern California
2025 Zonal Avenue
Los Angeles, CA 90033
(213) 342-1259

Georgia
James R. Eckman, M.D.
Department of Medicine
Emory University School of Medicine
69 Butler Street, NE
Atlanta, GA 30303
(404) 616-3572

Massachusetts
Lillian E.C. McMahon, M.D.
Boston City Hospital
818 Harrison Avenue, FGH-2
Boston, MA 02118
(617) 534-5727

New York
Sergio Piomelli, M.D.
College of Physicians & Surgeons
Columbia University
630 West 168 Street
New York, NY 10032
(212) 305-5808

Ronald L. Nagel, M.D.
Montefiore Hospital Medical Center — Rosenthal Main
111 East 210 Street
Bronx, NY 10467
(212) 920-6310

North Carolina
Wendell F. Rosse, M.D.
Duke University Medical Center
Box 3934 Morris Building
Durham, NC 27710
(919) 684-3724

Pennsylvania
Kwaku Ohene-Frempong, M.D.
The Children's Hospital of Philadelphia
34th Street & Civic Center Boulevard
Philadelphia, PA 19104
(215) 590-3423

Tennessee
Ernest A. Turner, M.D.
Department of Pediatrics
Meharry Medical College
1005 D.B. Todd Jr. Boulevard
Nashville, TN 37208
(615) 327-6763

2) The Bureau of Maternal and Child Health funds the **Council of Regional Networks for Genetic Services (CORN)**. CORN is a federation of the country's ten Regional Genetic Networks, the Alliance of Genetic Support Groups, and the national sickle cell programs. CORN coordinates national genetic services and is especially concerned with the public health aspects of genetics and the delivery of genetic services. One CORN committee is dedicated to sickle cell and other hemoglobin diseases. This committee is concerned about the qualifications for sickle cell counselors, and,

like all CORN members, is interested in developing ways to provide genetic services to underserved populations and to address unmet needs.

CORN's ten regional groups and their coordinators (as of 1994) are as follows:

GENES (New York, Puerto Rico, Virgin Islands)
Genetics Network of the Empire State, Puerto Rico, & the Virgin Islands
WCL&R — Room E 229
PO Box 509
Albany, NY 12201-0509
(518) 473-8036
Karen Greendale, M.A.

GLaRGG (Minnesota, Wisconsin, Illinois, Indiana, Ohio, Michigan)
Great Lakes Regional Genetics Group
328 Waisman Center
1500 Highland Avenue
Madison, WI 53705-2280
(608) 265-2907
Louise Elbaum

GPGSN (N. Dakota, S. Dakota, Nebraska, Kansas, Oklahoma, Iowa, Missouri, Arkansas)
Great Plains Genetics Service Network
Division of Medical Genetics
Department of Pediatrics
University of Iowa
Iowa City, IA 52242-1038
(319) 356-4860
Delores Nesbitt, Ph.D.

MARHGN (Pennsylvania, New Jersey, Delaware, Maryland, Washington, D.C., Virginia, W. Virginia)
Mid-Atlantic Regional Human Genetics Network
C/O Family Planning Council
260 South Broad Street, Suite 1900
Philadelphia, PA 19102-3865
(215) 985-6760
Gail Chiarrello, M.C.P.

MSRGSN (Montana, Wyoming, Utah, Arizona, Colorado, New Mexico)
Mountain States Regional Genetic Services Network
Colorado Department of Health
FCHS-MAS-A4
4300 Cherry Creek Drive South
Denver, CO 80222-1530
(303) 692-2423
Joyce Hooker

NERGG (Maine, New Hampshire, Vermont, Massachusetts, Connecticut, Rhode Island)
New England Regional Genetics Group
PO Box 670
Mt. Desert, ME 04660-0670
(207) 288-2704
Joseph Robinson, M.P.H.

PacNoRGG (Washington, Oregon, Idaho, Alaska)
Pacific Northwest Regional Genetics Group
Oregon Health Sciences University
CDRC—Clinical Services Building
901 East 18th Avenue
Eugene, OR 97403
(503) 346-2610
Kerry Silvey, M.A.

PSRGN (California, Nevada, Hawaii)
Pacific Southwest Regional Genetics Network
Department of Health Services
2151 Berkeley Way, Annex 4
Berkeley, CA 94704-9802
(510) 540-2696
Melinda Lassman, M.A., M.S.

SERGG (Kentucky, Tennessee, N. Carolina, S. Carolina, Louisiana,
Mississippi, Alabama, Georgia, Florida)
Southeastern Regional Genetics Group
Emory University School of Medicine
Pediatrics/Medical Genetics
2040 Ridgewood Road
Atlanta, GA 30322-4870
(404) 727-5844
Mary Rose Lane

TEXGENE (Texas)
Texas Genetics Program Coordinator
Bureau of Women and Children
Texas Department of Health
1100 West 49th Street
Austin, TX 78756-3199
(512) 458-7700
William Moore, M.H.A.

The State Genetic Services Coordinators (as of 1994) in alphabetical or-
der by state are as follows:

State Genetics and Hemoglobinopathies
Bureau of Family Health Services
Alabama Department of Public Health
434 Monroe Street
Montgomery, **Alabama** 36130
(205) 242-5760
Mary Ross

Genetics Coordinator
1231 Gambell Street, Room 313
Anchorage, **Alaska** 99501
(907) 274-3636
Christy Leblond, M.S.

Genetics Coordinator
Office of Women's and Children's Health
Arizona Department of Health
1740 West Adams, Room 200
Phoenix, **Arizona** 85007
(602) 542-1880
Dorris Evans-Gates

Genetics Program Coordinator
State of Arkansas
4815 West Markham, Slot 17
Little Rock, **Arkansas** 72205
(501) 661-2189
Pam Ashcraft, R.N.

Genetics Program Director
University of Arkansas Medical School,
Slot 506
4301 West Markham
Little Rock, **Arkansas** 72205
(501) 686-8338
Becky Butler, L.C.S.W.

Genetics Disease Branch
California State Department of Health Services
2152 Berkeley Way, Annex 4
Berkeley, **California** 94704-1011
(510) 540-2552
George C. Cunningham, M.D., M.P.H.

Mountain States Regional Genetics Network
FCHS-MA-A4
4300 Cherry Creek Drive, South
Denver, **Colorado** 80222-1530
(303) 692-2423
Joyce Hooker

Bureau of Community Health
State Department of Health Services
150 Washington Street
Hartford, **Connecticut** 06106
(203) 566-1143
Gretchen Landenburger, M.S.

Genetic Services Program
District of Columbia Bureau of Maternal and Child Services
1660 L Street, NW
Washington, **D.C.** 20036
(202) 673-6673
Jill Shuger, Sc.M.

Office of Genetic Services
Division of Public Health
Jesse S. Cooper Memorial Building
Dover, **Delaware** 19903
(302) 739-4786
Nancy Oyerly, R.N., M.S.

Prevention/Screening/Perinatal Unit
Children's Medical Services
1317 Winewood Boulevard
Tallahassee, **Florida** 32399
(904) 488-1465
Mittie Moffett, R.N., M.S.

Genetics Program Manager
Georgia Department of Human Resources
2600 Skyland Drive
Atlanta, **Georgia** 30319
(404) 679-0541
Mary Ann Henson, R.N., M.S.N.

PSRGN Genetics Coordinator—Hawaii
Kapiolani Medical Center
1319 Punahou Street, No. 535
Honolulu, **Hawaii** 96826
(808) 973-8795
Jana Hall, Ph.D.

Genetic Services Program Manager
Bureau of Laboratories
Idaho Department of Health and Welfare
2220 Old Penitentiary Road
Boise, **Idaho** 83712
(208) 334-2235
Mary Jane Webb

Genetic Program Coordinator
Division of Family Health
Illinois Department of Public Health
535 West Jefferson Street
Springfield, **Illinois** 62761
(217) 784-5992
Sydney Kling, R.N., M.A.

Division of Maternal and Child Health
Indiana State Department of Health
202 North John Street
Arcadia, **Indiana** 46430
(317) 633-0354
Taara Vanmeter, M.S.

State Genetics Coordinator
Regional Genetic Consultation Service
2605 JCP, 200 Hawkins Drive
Iowa City, **Iowa** 52242-1083
(800) 260-2065; (319) 356-2674
Jean Anderson, R.N., M.A., C.P.N.P.

Coordinator Genetic Services
Kansas Department of Health
Landon State Office
900 Southwest Jackson Street
Room 1005 North
Topeka, **Kansas** 66612-1290
(913) 296-1316
Carolyn Domingo, R.N., M.S.

Genetic Program Administrator
Pediatric Services Branch
Department of Health Services
Division of Maternal and Child Health
275 East Main Street
Frankfort, **Kentucky** 40621
(502) 564-2154
Darlene Goodrich

Administrator, Genetic Diseases Program
Department of Health and Hospitals
Office of Public Health, Room 308
New Orleans, **Louisiana** 70160
(504) 568-5070
Charles Myers, M.S.W.

Division of Maternal and Child Health
Department of Human Services
State House, Station 11
151 Capital Street
Augusta, **Maine** 04333
(207) 289-3311
Cheryl Dicara, B.S.W.

Division of Hereditary Disorders
Maryland Department of Health & Mental Hygiene
PO Box 13528
Baltimore, **Maryland** 21203
(301) 225-6730
Susan R. Panny, M.D.

Genetics Education Coordinator
Department of Public Health
150 Tremont Street
Boston, **Massachusetts** 02111
(617) 727-5121
Robin Blatt, M.P.H.

State Department of Public Health
3500 North Logan Street
Lansing, **Michigan** 48909
(517) 335-8938
William Young, Ph.D.

Human Genetics Unit
PO Box 9441
Minneapolis, **Minnesota** 55440
(612) 623-5268
Malcolm Jenkins, Ph.D.

Mississippi State Department of Health
Genetic Screening Program
PO Box 1700
Jackson, **Mississippi** 39215-1700
(601) 960-7619
Daniel Bender, M.H.S.

Associate Bureau Chief for Genetic Services
Bureau for Special Health Care Needs
Missouri Department of Health
1730 East Elm Street
Jefferson City, **Missouri** 65102
(314) 751-6246
N. Aurita Prince Caldwell, M.Ed.

Shodair Children's Hospital
Montana Medical Genetic Program
Box 5539
Helena, **Montana** 59604
(406) 444-7530
John Opitz, M.D.

Director, Maternal and Child Health
Nebraska State Health Department
301 Centennial Mall South
Lincoln, **Nebraska** 68509-5007
(402) 471-2907
Monica Seeland

Perinatal Coordinator
Nevada Division of Health
505 East King, Room 205
Carson City, **Nevada** 89710
(702) 687-4885
Eileen Coulombe

Genetic Services
Bureau of Special Medical Services
6 Hazen Drive
Concord, **New Hampshire** 03301
(603) 271-4533
Susan Z. Berg

Coordinator of Disorders and Genetics
New Jersey State Department of Health, SCHS\SPSP
363 West State Street, CN 364
Trenton, **New Jersey** 08625-0364
(609) 983-1343
Lorra L. Hambach, M.P.H.

Program Manager, Child Health Section
New Mexico Department of Health
1190 Saint Francis Drive
Santa Fe, **New Mexico** 87502
(505) 827-2353
C. Holly Nyerges, M.S.N., C.P.N.P.

Director, New York State Genetics Program
Laboratory of Human Genetics
Wadsworth Center for Laboratories and Research
New York State Department of Health
PO Box 509
Albany, **New York** 12201-0509
(518) 473-1993
Ken Pass, Ph.D.

Coordinator, CORN
Cornell University Medical College
1300 York Avenue
Genetics, Box 53
New York, **New York** 10021
(212) 746-3475
Karin S. Stern, R.N., Dr. P.H.

Co-Director, Division of Human Genetics
The New York Hospital
525 East 68th Street
New York, **New York** 10021
(212) 746-1496
Jessica G. Davis, M.D.

Program Manager
Division of Maternal and Child Health
Genetic Health Care and Newborn Screening
PO Box 27687
Raleigh, **North Carolina** 27611-7687
(919) 715-3420
Elizabeth Moore, M.S.S.W.

State Genetics Coordinator
Medical Genetics Division
University of North Dakota Medical School
501 Columbia Road
Grand Forks, **North Dakota** 58203
(701) 777-4243
Mary Ebertowski

Genetics Program Coordinator
Early Intervention Unit
Ohio Department of Health
246 North High Street, 4th Floor
Columbus, **Ohio** 43266-0118
(614) 644-8389
Debra Wright, R.N.C., B.S.N.

Genetics Section
Oklahoma State Department of Health
1000 Northeast 10th Street
Oklahoma City, **Oklahoma** 73152
(405) 271-6617
Shari Kinney

State Genetic Services Coordinator
CDRC — Clinical Services Building
901 East 18th Street
Eugene, **Oregon** 97403
(503) 346-2610
Kerry Silvey, M.A.

Director, Genetics and SIDS Program
Division of Maternal and Child Health
Department of Health
PO Box 90
Harrisburg, **Pennsylvania** 17108
(717) 783-8143
Jana Burdge

University Pediatric Hospital
University of Puerto Rico Medical School
GPO Box 5067
San Juan, **Puerto Rico** 00936
(809) 754-7410
Enid Rivera, M.D.

Division of Family Health
Department of Health
3 Capitol Hill
Providence, **Rhode Island** 02908
(401) 277-2312
Peter Simon, M.D.

Bureau of Maternal and Child Health
Division of Children's Rehabilitative Services
2600 Bull Street
Columbia, **South Carolina** 29201
(803) 737-4050
Marie Thompson

University of South Dakota School of Medicine
1011 11th Street
Rapid City, **South Dakota** 57701
(605) 394-5110
Carol Strom, M.S.

Director, Tennessee Genetics Program
Tennessee Department of Health and Environment
525 Cordell Hull Building
100 9th Avenue, North
Nashville, **Tennessee** 37247-4701
(615) 741-7335
Janet Ulm

Genetics Program Coordinator
Bureau of Maternal and Child Health
Texas Department of Health
1100 West 49th Street
Austin, **Texas** 78756-3199
(512) 458-7700
William E. Moore, M.H.A.

State Genetics Coordinator
Division of Medical Genetics
University of Utah Medical Center
50 N. Medical Drive
Salt Lake City, **Utah** 84132
(801) 581-8943
John Carey, M.D.

Division of Public Health Analysis and Policy
Vermont Department of Health
212 Battery Street
Burlington, **Vermont** 05402
(802) 863-7606
Ellen Thompson, R.D., M.S.

Genetics Coordinator — MARGN
Virginia State Department of Health
1500 East Main Street
Richmond, **Virginia** 23218
(804) 786-7367
Arlethia Rogers, R.N.

Department of Health
48 Sugar Estates
United States **Virgin Islands** 00802
(809) 774-1746
C. Patricia Penn, Genetics Program Coordinator
Mavis Matthews, M.D., M.P.H., Director,
Division of Maternal and Child Health

Office of Maternal/Infant Health and Genetics
Genetic Services Coordinator
Department of Social and Health Services
1704 N.E. 150th Street, K17-8
Seattle, **Washington** 98155-7226
(206) 368-4471
Debra Lochner Doyle, M.S.

Genetics Program Coordinator
Bureau of Public Health
1414 East Washington Avenue, Room 96
Madison, **Wisconsin** 53703-3044
(608) 266-8904
Gladys Kitson

Director, Genetics Evaluation and Counseling
West Virginia University Medical Center
Morgantown, **West Virginia** 26506
(304) 293-7331
Mary Beth Hummel, M.D.

Wyoming Genetic Program
Department of Health
461 Hathaway Building
Cheyenne, **Wyoming** 82002
(307) 777-7166
Larry Goodmay, M.S., M.B.A.

The **Alliance of Genetic Support Groups** is a consortium of about 250 consumer groups that provide psychosocial support to people with all kinds of genetic diseases and their families. It is a resource for consumers seeking genetic support groups as well as for genetic counselors, nurses, social workers, physicians, researchers, educators, students, librarians, and the media. The Alliance publishes a monthly newsletter. Its address is 35 Wisconsin Circle, Suite 440, Chevy Chase, Maryland 20815-7015. The toll-free number is 800-336-GENE.

Planned Parenthood, a not-for-profit organization, runs almost 1,000 family-planning clinics in the United States. They have a sliding fee scale, so people are billed according to their ability to pay. If there is a Planned Parenthood clinic within 50 miles of your home, you can make an appointment there by calling 1-800-230-PLAN. If there is not a clinic within 50 miles, try your local telephone directory or call the Planned Parenthood Federation of America at (212) 541-7800.

Notes

1. There is an exception to this. In the female, the two sex chromosomes (designated XX) constitute a pair, but in the male, the two sex chromosomes (designated XY) do not. Since males have only one-of-a-kind sex chromosomes, the genes on them are not paired.

2. Actually, about one or two such people in every thousand do have one blue eye and one brown eye. Eye color inheritance is not fully understood, and it is more complicated than this discussion implies.

3. Linus Pauling, who died as this book went to press, was the only person to ever win two unshared Nobel Prizes. He was awarded the Chemistry Prize in 1954, and, as an activist for world disarmament, was awarded the Peace Prize in 1962.

4. L. Pauling, H.A. Itano, S.J. Singer, and I.C. Wells, "Sickle Cell Anemia: A Molecular Disease," *Science* 110 (1949): 543-48.

5. R. Lebby, "Case of Absence of the Spleen," *Southern Journal of Medical Pharmacology* 1 (1846): 481-83.

6. J.B. Herrick, "Peculiar Elongated and Sickle-Shaped Red Blood Corpuscles in a Case of Severe Anemia," *Archives of Internal Medicine* 6 (1910): 517-21.

7. Out of respect for privacy, patient names are not published in medical reports. Hence, Dr. Noel's identity was not known prior to the recent publication of a follow-up story of the patient who was the subject of the first sickle cell disease report in Western medical literature: T.L. Savitt and M.F. Goldberg, "Herrick's 1910 Case Report of Sickle Cell Anemia: The Rest of the Story," *Journal of the American Medical Association* 261 (1985): 266-71. Noel's name was used in that publication by permission of his step-grandnephew.

8. Charles Darwin was horrified that among humans, too, the strong (fittest) survived at the expense of the weak. He detested slavery. "It makes one's blood boil, yet heart tremble, to think that we Englishmen and our American descendants, with their boastful cry of liberty, have been and are so guilty...," he wrote. Darwin's father-in-law, Josiah Wedgwood (the china manufacturer), was one of the earliest antislavery activists

in England. (A. Moorehead, *Darwin and the Beagle*, New York: Harper and Row, 1969.)

9. *Evolution* is the continuous process by which living things adapt to their environment. Evolution produces new species, new races, and, in the shorter term, new strains. The flu virus, for example, evolves into a different strain almost every year, and that is why we must get a new vaccination each flu season. The use of antibiotics has brought about the evolution of drug-resistant organisms. The resurgence of tuberculosis in the United States is due to the adaptation of the tubercle bacillus to the drugs that were designed to kill it. Evolution is an ongoing process, so there are always examples around to study.

10. A slave trade existed in Africa long before the Europeans came, and the Muslims were its primary supporters. The principal slaveholders were the Mohammedan kingdoms of North and West Africa (among their purchases were women and eunuchs for Muslim harems), Morocco, Egypt, and Zanzibar, and the Christian kingdom of Abyssinia. There was also slavery in Negro kingdoms such as Uganda and Benin, where many slaves were sacrificed in religious ceremonies. Moreover, throughout Africa, warring tribes kept their captives as slaves and invaded neighboring areas to capture women. Prior to the Portuguese era, however, slaves were not shipped across the Atlantic. (T. Buxton, "Slavery," *Encyclopedia Britannica*, 1951.)

11. R. Nagel, "Sickle Cell: Model for Medicine's Future," *Einstein* (Summer 1993): 11-12.

12. M. Wintrobe, "Milestones on the Path of Progress," in *Blood, Pure and Eloquent*, M. Wintrobe, ed., McGraw-Hill, 1980: Chapter 1.

13. The milligram is a measure of weight in the *metric system*. There are 28,350 milligrams in an ounce. Other metric system units that may be more familiar are the kilometer, which measures length, and the liter, which measures volume.

14. Acute Pain Management Panel, 1992, *Acute Pain Management: Operative or Medical Procedures and Trauma: Clinical Practice Guideline*, AHCPR Pub. No. 92-0032, Rockville, MD: Agency for Health Care Policy and Research, U.S. Public Health Service.

15. D.J. Weatherall, *The New Genetics and Clinical Practice*, 3rd edition, Oxford University Press, 1991.

16. If the remaining cells were permitted to develop into a fetus, the fetus would never miss the cell that had been removed. In fact, every one of the cells at this early stage of development could develop into its own fetus, and they would all be identical "twins."

17. Clinical trials test new treatments on groups of volunteers. The volunteers know the treatment is experimental, and they give "informed consent" before being entered into the trial. Early trials ask two basic questions: (1) At what dose, if any, does the treatment seem to help the disease, and (2) What are the harmful effects of the treatment?

18. J. Watson, "The Significance of the Paucity of Sickle Cells in Newborn Negro Infants," *American Journal of Medical Science* 215 (1948): 419-23.

19. J.L. Touraine, "In Utero Transplantation of Fetal Liver Stem Cells in Humans," *Blood Cells* 17 (1991): 379-87.

20. Gene therapy does not change a person's chances of having sickle cell children. Treated individuals would not transmit their transplanted genes to the next generation because the gametes would not have received copies of them. Only marrow cells would receive the good hemoglobin genes.

Index